The Expectant Dairy Cow

Julian Hill BSc (Hons), PhD
Writtle College, Chelmsford, Essex, CM1 3RR,
United Kingdom

and

Anthony H. Andrews BVetMed, PhD, MRCVS, MBIAC
Acorn House, Mardley Hill, Welwyn, Hertfordshire,
AL6 0TT, United Kingdom

Chalcombe Publications

First published in the United Kingdom by
Chalcombe Publications
Church Lane, Welton, Lincoln, LN2 3LT,
United Kingdom

ISBN 0948617 42 X

Cover photo : Holstein Friesian cow eight months pregnant with her second calf.

Printed by Ruddocks Printers Ltd Lincoln.

CONTENTS

Page

PREFACE

Why is the expectant cow overlooked ? Several reasons can be cited. The assumption that the cow with the lowest requirement for nutrients compared with other stages of the lactation cycle is of lower priority seems nonsensical, but this view has prevailed for many years. If poor management of the cow occurs during late pregnancy, a reduction in the level of colostrum and its quality, a reduction in the yield of milk and/or milk constituents, an increase in metabolic and nutritional disorders and possibly impaired fertility may result with loss in income to the farmer. Secondly, but probably more important, is the potential reduction in the efficiency of reproduction of the cow as a result of anoestrus in the ensuing lactation, a decline in conception rate or the production of a non-viable calf.

Recently, the nutrition of the cow in late pregnancy has received more attention from research workers, leading to significant findings which have changed our perceptions of how to feed and manage the cow during the transition from pregnancy to lactation.

IMPORTANT NOTE:
The aim of this book is to provide practical information, in a user-friendly fashion, on the scientific advances in the management of the pregnant and dry cow. While every effort has been made to ensure that the content of this book is correct, the authors cannot be held responsible for any errors, omissions or commissions. Where any rations are considered, formulated or utilised, it is essential to check the efficacy and adequacy of the ration with your nutrition adviser or another suitable source. Where any therapy or control measure is suggested it is essential to check this with your veterinary surgeon or other suitable source. Any preparation mentioned must only be used following full consultation of any data sheet produced for that product and must only be used in the manner indicated by that data sheet.

J Hill   A H Andrews   March 2000

Chapter 1
INTRODUCTION

1.1 What is the dry period?

The dry period can best be described as a short break or "rest" between lactations. The duration of the period is usually seven to nine weeks (50 to 60 days). The time is essential for several reasons related to the health of the cow, the unborn calf and the stress of the following lactation. First, it is the period when the cow prepares herself for the sustained production of milk by ensuring her reserves of energy, protein and minerals are optimal. It is well known that during the first six to eight weeks of lactation that the cow cannot consume enough food to maintain a high yield of milk and therefore the cow has to mobilise body reserves ("milking off her back") to maintain production (see Chapters 5 and 6).

The second reason for the dry period is that the cow has to provide for the ever increasing demand for energy and protein by the unborn calf. The mechanisms of control and role of nutrition for this vital function are outlined in Chapters 2, 5 and 6.

The third reason for the dry period is to allow for the repair, growth and development of milk secretory tissue in the udder. If the period of rest between lactations is too short, it is logical that the repair and growth of new milk producing tissue in the udder may well be reduced or impaired (Chapter 3).

Finally, the dry period, especially its last 14 days, is a period when the digestive system of the cow has to adapt from a low to a high plane of nutrition. This critical period and imminent change in ration must be considered carefully to ensure that nutrient utilisation in the subsequent lactation is optimal.

All of the above factors can be manipulated to a greater or lesser extent by carefully controlling the nutrition of the cow during late lactation (that is after 250 days in milk) and the dry period.

1.2 Duration of the dry period

The normal length of the dry period is about 50 to 60 days. This duration of time has, it seems, been determined by the economics of milk production rather than by the health and welfare of the cow. Maximum income realised per lactation relies on the performance of the cow during lactation (the efficiency of conversion of feed to milk constituents), the efficiency of reproduction and the susceptibility or not to disease. Reproductive efficiency is therefore a key factor in determining the dry period. The calving interval is defined as the period from the birth of a calf to the birth of the next calf and the calving interval can be used as a method of determining the economic and reproductive efficiency of a herd.

It has been shown by many economic and nutrition studies that the maximum income returned from milk sales in relation to total feed cost occurs with calving intervals of 330 to 395 days in length, that is 11 to 13 months of milk production. If however, the mean dry period is 56 days (eight weeks), the time in milk will range from 275 to 340 days with a mean of 310 days. Therefore, to achieve a 12-month calving interval for all cows in a herd is difficult (if not impossible) even under exceptional management regimes. Inevitably, if a strict regime of 12 months calving interval is to be maintained a number of good milking cows would be sold or culled. Is this good economic sense? Second, this philosophy may not be correct for very high yielding cows where lifetime milk production could be a better measure and one which takes into consideration the welfare of the cow.

An alternative strategy to ensure maximum milk sales per annum would be to shorten the dry period to reduce feed costs when the cow is not producing milk. This is not a good idea for reasons that are, or will become, obvious. Both strategies have a detrimental effect on the welfare of the cow. First, it is known that very short periods of rest between lactations (less than six weeks) reduce the yield of milk in the next lactation. This may reflect an insufficient period of time for the cow to repair existing milk producing tissue in the udder and also insufficient time for the cow to build up body reserves that will be utilised in the next lactation. The issues that arise from reducing the level of feed during the dry period and/or having a too a short a dry period will be developed in detail in Chapters 5 and 6.

In the United Kingdom, annual milk quota restricts the level of production and may in some instances lead to producers considering drying cows off earlier than 300 days of lactation. Extending the dry period can have several detrimental effects on the cow, for instance excessive condition (too fat) at calving reducing the voluntary intake of the cow in the next lactation, fatty liver and other nutritional and metabolic disorders, and potentially reduced fertility.

If, during lactation, an event occurs which reduces milk yield (for example, mastitis; Chapter 3) and/or the lactating tissue of the udder is damaged to a point when milk yield is compromised, an extended dry period may occur. This scenario is probably more common than is first thought and the management of the cow after the point of production failure is extremely difficult. The cow must be fed at a level which prevents her from becoming over-fat and therefore prone to metabolic disorders before and after the next calving. More detail on these issues will be discussed in Chapters 4, 5 and 6. If the dry period is extended deliberately (for example if the herd is over milk quota), the potential increase in milk yield in the next lactation is unlikely to offset the extra cost of feeding the cow during the extended dry period. It may well mean that the herd is not realising its maximum potential financially. Control of overall milk production from the herd to maximise financial performance may also be achieved by other strategies, for instance acquisition of quota, reduction in level of feeding in mid and late lactation.

1.3 Impact of extended lactations and "elite" herds

The average yield of milk produced by Holstein-Friesian cows in the UK is 6028 kg per 305 days. If these cows are considered average, elite cows may yield twice the average lactation yield. The physiological and metabolic "strain" on these cows are enormous and therefore very precise management regimes have to be applied during the period of milk production. It has been suggested earlier, that poor management of cows during the dry period, especially the last 14 days of pregnancy, can reduce substantially milk production in the subsequent lactation. Therefore the development of elite herds (lactation yields of over 12000 litres per cow) poses a series of challenges to the farmer, the veterinary surgeon and the nutritionist. In herds such as this, maximum income is not achieved during months 11 to 13 but from months 15 to 18 of lactation. Production indicators therefore need to be changed from yield per 305 day lactation to life-time yield and yield per lactation year. Often this procedure is done retrospectively. The extended lactation may place further stresses on the cow and the udder. Does the increase in milk yield over the extended lactation mean the dry period has to be extended? An extension of the dry period may, in theory, lead to animals entering the next production phase with greater reserves of body tissues that can be mobilised but the method to achieve this is far from being completely developed and there is no evidence to date that this approach gives a higher return in income. The current methods used to feed cows during the dry period are not usually suitable for elite cows. A recent study in the UK suggested that increased care and attention to detail during the dry period must be taken for elite cows. When elite cows were managed in groups of "normal" cows, an increase in the incidence of milk fever (hypocalcaemia) has been observed.

The key issue to be addressed is the interaction between yield per day and duration of lactation. In general, three times a day milking regimes are essential in the management of "elite" cows. Secretory cells in the alveoli of the udder will only respond to stimulation (for example changes in the pattern of milking) if nutrients are present in sufficient quantities. However, the greater the degree of stimulation of the secretory cells the greater the risk of damage to the secretory tissue of the udder and therefore a greater risk of disease. If the cow cannot supply adequate nutrients to the mammary gland during early lactation (weeks 0 to 4), yield potential will not be reached. Thus she needs to start lactation with as high a dry matter intake as possible - by offering high quality rations. If not there may be too many cows being culled young and therefore lifetime yield must be examined in the case of "elite" cows.

The nutrition of the "elite" cow during the dry period must therefore be accurate and will probably be different to that given to the average cow (a six to eight week dry period is suggested for normal yielding cows but may well need to be increased for elite cows). The diet must ensure nutrients are targeted to the udder to allow the udder to be repaired and fully functional for the rigours of the next lactation. Body reserves must be manipulated thus allowing the cow to maintain the maximum rate of release of nutrients during the period of greatest lactational stress (that is when the food intake of the cow is too low to maintain milk production in early lactation). The body reserves must also supply the correct nutrients during the period of nutritional deficit.

Finally, the voluntary intake of the cow must be maximised during early lactation and therefore special diets may be required in the last two weeks of the dry period to "condition" the rumen to the production ration. This will be discussed in more detail in Chapter 5.

Chapter 2

PREGNANCY AND FOETAL PHYSIOLOGY

2.0 Introduction

Poor reproductive efficiency is costing the UK dairy sector approximately £200 million per year. There are various reasons for the poor efficiency of many herds, for instance the low rate of detection of oestrus, problems associated with the nutrition and management of the lactating cow early in the production cycle leading to high embryo mortality and potentially poor management of the dry cow. This chapter examines these issues and the role of the placenta and the development of the foetus in relation to nutrient supply.

2.1 Ovarian function and follicle production

Follicle production and development is an important factor affecting the efficiency of reproduction of the dairy cow. Several thousand primordial follicles are produced as a result of ovarian development *in uteru*, however only 0.1 to 0.2% of these primordial follicles will mature to be able to develop an ovum and hence facilitate reproduction. The factors which control the further development of primordial follicles are poorly understood. However the supply of nutrients to the developing embryo must be a key factor in understanding the reproductive efficiency of the cow. Therefore nutritional management of the lactating and dry cow is important in the development of follicle primordia.

The control of follicular growth and development is the interaction between the ovary and the hypothalamus-pituitary axis, non gonadotropin hormones (e.g. growth hormones, insulin and IGF) and intra-ovarian control mechanisms including the control of fibroblasts, epidermal growth factor and various transforming growth factors.

Follicle growth and development to a mature ovum occurs in a wave-like pattern during the ovarian cycle. Two or three waves of recruitment (5 to 7 follicles of >5mm) results in the growth of one ovum (15 mm dominance) which remains for 2 to 3 days before atresia (degeneration). If however the development of the dominant ovum coincides with luteolysis, the follicle matures and is released as a result of ovulation. Dominance is potentially controlled by a decrease in follicle stimulating hormone (FSH) and the direct inhibition of other follicles. Management of nutrient supply during several stages of the production cycle has to be monitored carefully to ensure that follicular growth and development to a mature ovum are not compromised. If follicular development and growth are compromised by poor or inappropriate nutrition, the calving interval of the cow will be extended and income lost. The key to high efficiency of reproduction is the balance between the animal factors affecting ovulation and oocyte receptiveness and the timing of insemination, whether artificial or by natural service.

Even though the requirements for follicular development are low (about 3 MJ of metabolisable energy per day), the potential impact of severe negative energy balance in early lactation leads to impaired fertility, by reducing the likelihood of an early resumption of ovarian activity. This is especially noticeable in "elite" herds. Lead feeding in late pregnancy may actually make the situation worse as cows may enter lactation too fat and therefore their voluntary intake may be reduced during the critical period of 0 to 42 days of milk production. Restriction of energy supply during the period of oocyte (egg) development leads to the formation of oocytes from small follicles and may reduce the fertilisation rate. However the number of oocytes recovered is lower in cattle fed adequate supplies of energy and therefore, it seems that nutritional effects on reproduction can also occur at a stage prior to ovulation.

2.2 Oestrus detection

The detection of oestrus activity is important for a successful reproductive strategy in a herd. It has been estimated that approximately 50% of fertility problems with dairy cows are associated with poor detection of "heat", or oestrus. The economic implications of poor oestrus detection is about £2.75 to £3.00 per cow per day, if not served after observed oestrus. If artificial insemination is to be used as the preferred method of genetic improvement of dairy cattle within a herd, accurate detection of oestrus is essential and any method of improving the rate of detection should be implemented as part of a herd management strategy. The period from calving to first service (the waiting period) should be about seven weeks. To achieve a 365 days calving interval, only a maximum of 2 cycles can be observed after the waiting period if a rigid pattern of calving is to be maintained. In practice many cows have a calving interval of greater than 365 days and the pattern of calving is related to the accuracy of heat detection.

Two key methods of determining the reproductive efficiency of a dairy herd are the submission rate and the rate of return. The submission rate is a measure of how many cows and heifers are served in a 21-day period compared to the total number of cows available for service in the herd. Submission rates should be about 80%. The rate of return is the number of cows returning to oestrus within 12 to 30 days of the previous detection and service. The average level of heat detection is about 55% and therefore with only 50% of cows getting pregnant to any service a significant slippage in calving pattern can occur. It is also interesting to note that estimated rates of detection of heat are higher in herds of greater than 100 cows (55 to 59%) than in herds of less than 100 cows (44 to 46%) but no reduction in accuracy of detection was observed.

The normal length of the oestrus cycle is 21 days but the range can be from 12 to 30 days. The typical pattern of behaviour associated with oestrus lasts for two to three days and is characterised by:

Aggressive bunting and rubbing (from -48 hours to +18 hours of oestrus)
Investigatory sniffing around the tail head (from -24 hours to +15 hours of oestrus)
Chin resting (-18 hours to about +12 hours of oestrus)
Orientation to mount (about -12 hours to +12 hours of oestrus)
Disorientated mounting (-6 hours to + 12 hours of oestrus)
Standing to be mounted (+0 hours to +12 hours of oestrus)

The latter pattern of behaviour is the critical sign of oestrus and lasts between 8 and 12 hours. The best time for artificial insemination occurs between 6 and 30 hours after oestrus, when concentrations of luteinising hormone are at their maximum. Ovulation occurs generally 24 to 30 hours after the start of the behavioural change to standing to be mounted and is spread over a period of about 10 hours. It is important to ensure insemination occurs at least 8 to 10 hours before ovulation as the time taken for sperm to reach the oviduct and undergo capacitation is about 6 to 10 hours. Capacitation is the process of imbibation of secretions from the cows reproductive tract and hence conferring "fertility". Fertilisation of the released ovum can then occur in the oviduct. Oestrus behaviour can be observed in cattle that are in-calf (8 to 10%) and therefore it is important to record accurately all oestrus events over a number of years.

The best time to observe oestrus activity in cattle is at dawn or dusk in grazing cows or at mid afternoon or night in housed cows. Herds observed after 10 pm at night had higher levels of detection of oestrous (55-75%) compared to herds with no observations made after 8 pm (46%). Other times when oestrus activity can be observed are when cows are not being fed or milked but "stirred-up" for some reason. The degree of activity observed is affected by the number of cows in active oestrus, the ambient environment and conditions of housing.

Heat detection is difficult when cows are lame, oestrus starts during late evening or the night, when cows are already showing oestrus activity or are high yielding and losing weight rapidly.

There are many aids to detecting oestrus, for instance calendar systems to predict next oestrus, milk progesterone monitoring, tail paint, pastes or marking crayons, Kamars, closed circuit TV, pedometers or modified or treated animals (vasectomised bulls, testosterone-treated females or androgenised steers). These methods can on average improve detection by 6 to 10% compared with herds not using aids to detection. However the most important factor in oestrus detection is the maintenance of accurate records and a routine to observe cows regularly during the critical periods of the day. In herds observing cows four times a day, greater efficiency of detection of oestrus was observed compared with herds observed three times or less (61% vs. 52%, respectively).

The Management of Insemination by Routine Analysis (MOIRA) system is based on monitoring progesterone concentrations in milk. MOIRA can help to identify cows which have abnormal patterns of oestrus, thus facilitating veterinary examination and pharmacological treatment. It is also very useful in identifying cows returning to service. The system is based on a series of tests at weekly intervals to determine if the cow is cycling. The procedure starts 20 days post calving and the concentration of progesterone in the milk is thereafter noted as low (L), medium (M) or high (H). Patterns of anoestrus (LLL), cystic corpus luteum (HHH) or short cycling/follicular cysts (LHL) can be determined and used to determine pregnancy or use of pharmacological treatment. A pattern of HHH could however be an indication of pregnancy. The key to the success of the MOIRA system is that whilst it does not measure the actual concentration of progesterone circulating it does allow the monitoring of patterns of change.

2.3 Pregnancy, placenta function and foetal physiology

Under normal conditions where there are no nutritional stresses or health problems with the cow, the primary source of nutrients for the developing calf are derived from maternal reserves. Nutrients supplied to the developing calf are transported across and therefore regulated by the placenta. The placenta is the interface between the cow and her calf and therefore the development and maintenance of the placenta is very important for, not only the viability of the calf, but subsequent milk production.

2.3.1 Embryo development, placenta growth and metabolism

After fertilisation, the fertilised ovum travels down the oviduct into the uterus. During this period the fertilised ovum has undergone a number of cell divisions and by the 16-cell stage (the blastocyst), the conceptus is running low on endogenous reserves. The process of attachment and implantation of the blastocyst is therefore very important for its survival and a successful pregnancy. About 25% of embryos are lost during the first 3 weeks of life and the likely cause of embryo loss is the occurrence of luteolysis. Maintenance of progesterone output is essential in early pregnancy and therefore loss of the corpus luteum will lead to a loss in the mechanism of maternal recognition. The corpus luteum is also potentially controlled by luteal oxytocin and endometrial receptors. In early pregnancy the production of prostaglandin (PGF2α) is inhibited and no significant increases in numbers of endometrial oxytocin receptors occur as a result of the production of specific bovine embryo-derived interferons which prevent luteal regression.

In ruminants, distinct areas of projecting tissue (carcuncles, aglandular uterine mucosa) are located about half way between the cervix and the junction of the oviduct. These sites are the only places where successful attachment of the blastocyst can occur. The surface of the caruncle is covered with depressions known as crypts and the surface of the crypts are penetrated (but not fused) with foetal blood vessels in small villi after the process of implantation. The embryo enters the uterine horn about 4 to 5 days after fertilisation (the morula stage) and develops into the blastocyst (hollowing of the morula stage) at about Day 6 to 7. Hatching of the embryo from the zona pellucida occurs after about 10 days and elongation of the embryo starts. Maternal recognition of pregnancy occurs about 15 days after fertilisation and is a result of luteal function and the inhibition of luteolysis. Specific proteins (bovine interferon-α; IFN-α) are produced by the embryonic trophectoderm layer of the developing blastocyst. Expression of the protein ceases about Day 19 and attachment can occur. It has been suggested that embryo mortality occurring during Days 14 to 19 may be as a result of low production of IFN-α and therefore the onset of luteolysis. Pharmacological therapy to reduce embryo losses during early stages of recognition and attachment have been based on the use of gonadotrophic agents such as human chorionic gonadotrophin (hCG) or gonadotrophin releasing hormone (GnRH) or the use of progesterone analogues or interferons. These methods aim to reduce the incidence of failure of IFN-α secretion and therefore reducing luteolysis. However, they do not address the issues concerning the loss of embryos before Days 14 to 19 or the failure of fertilisation.

Early attachment of the embryo to the endometrium occurs at about Day 19 of development and the process of adhesion occurs after 22 days. Typically 66% of embryos are still viable after 19 days (attachment) but further losses can occur leading to a calving rate (number of calves born) of 55% at 280 days gestation. Once attachment has taken place, implantation of the conceptus occurs. The process of implantation is when the epithelium and endometrium (lining of the uterus) are penetrated by many cellular outgrowths developed by the conceptus. This process is the key to survival for the developing conceptus as it creates the continuum between the foetus and the mother. The incidence of embryo and foetal loss is also associated with lactation yield. Consistently higher incidences of early embryo loss occurred in herds of mean lactation yields of greater than 8500 l (15.0%) compared with herds of less than 5000 l (10.3%). Age of cow also can affect the incidence of embryo loss, however the differences between heifers (9.4%) and multiparous cows (10.7%) were relatively small.

Once the processes of attachment and implantation have been successful, the development of the placenta takes place. In many species, the link between the foetus and the mother is strong, with the majority of the link being the foetomaternal syncytium along the length of the uterus. Ruminants are different. Large areas of the placenta are not directly linked (a syncytia) but apposed (touching) to the endometrium. The close apposition between the foetus and the mother does not hinder the transfer of nutrients as there is close contact between the maternal blood system and the foetal circulatory system. This allows the transfer of nutrients from the mother to the developing calf and the removal of toxins produced by the calf.

As the placenta develops and grows, embryonic membranes are formed to develop a yolk sac. These membranes have an important role, the protection of the developing calf in the uterus. When these membranes are fully developed they form the amniotic sac. During the period of membrane formation, the placenta is growing rapidly and will develop many cotyledons (small protusions). Up to 150 cotyledons can be formed by the placenta of sheep or cows and are unique to animals where attachment of the placenta is limited to caruncles. The bovine placenta is made up of many small functional units known as placentomes. Each of these comprises a foetal cotyledon and a maternal caruncle.

The mature placenta is not fully functional until about 30 days after implantation. This does not mean that the placenta has reached its maximum size but it is able to support the transfer of nutrients from the cow to the foetus efficiently.

It is interesting to note that the processes of attachment and implantation, growth of the placenta and development of a viable pregnancy occur during the the first three months of lactation. The first ovarian activity after calving can occur as early as Day 14 of lactation. In practice cows are not served until at least 50 to 60 days after calving as the condition of the uterus and the nutritional status of the cow (negative energy balance) could impair conception. In fact if service is attempted, conception rates are low. Bear in mind the nutritional status of the cow. She is in early lactation, implantation and attachment are occurring at about day 65 to 70 and the potential impact of negative energy balance (that is milking off her back) could lead the cow to be under a great deal of metabolic and physiological stress.

There is a clear positive correlation between the severity of negative energy balance and the timing of first ovulation after calving. Ovulation does not occur until the negative energy balance is being reduced by increased intake of energy and a slow reduction in milk yield. Follicular competence is also related closely to the changes in negative energy balance with optimal competence occurring after the period of maximum negative energy balance.

The incidence of embryo loss has been shown to be higher in cows inseminated less than 50 days post partum (43%) compared with cows served approximately 60 days post partum (15 to 20%). It is therefore essential to ensure the cow does not lose condition too rapidly immediately after calving. This is achieved by correct feeding in the dry period thus ensuring the body reserves are optimal and can be mobilised. It is also essential that the ova produced for fertilisation have optimal reserves of energy and protein to allow cell division before attachment and implantation.

If the nutrition of the cow or heifer has been poor during the dry period, excessive negative energy balance will ensue, leading to metabolic and nutritional imbalances that will lead to adverse conditions for attachment and implantation thus leading to early embryo loss. In the worse-case scenario, anoestrous may occur after early embryo loss and therefore partial or complete cessation of reproductive performance. It has been noted in research in the USA, that lead feeding with fat supplements in late pregnancy may have the effect of shortening the period from calving to first ovulation. These issues are not related simply to an increase in supply of energy and will be discussed more fully in Chapters 5 and 6.

2.3.2 Confirming pregnancy in dairy cattle

Accurate confirmation of pregnancy and correct use of therapy can improve the reproductive efficiency of a dairy herd. The implementation of a herd management system such as MOIRA or the Knowledge Based System (KBS) can increase the profitability of animals by as much as £45 to £65 per cow after the third year of use.

Long-term systems may seem to be costly initially but are useful and economic so long as they are fully utilised by the farmer.

Rectal palpation has been used for many years as a method of diagnosing pregnancy and monitoring ovarian status. Accuracy of the method is however very dependent on skill of the veterinarian. Rectal palpation can also lead to failure of pregnancy, however the incidence of loss of embryo as a result is relatively low (1 to 2%).

The use of ultrasonography for pregnancy diagnosis and ovarian status has become increasing popular. The advent of real-time B-mode ultrasonography has allowed accurate studies of ovarian activity and determination of follicular dynamics. In conjunction with rectal palpation, ultrasonography is an important tool for pregnancy diagnosis.

2.3.3 Placenta function

The placenta is a highly complex organ, the interface between the cow and the developing calf. The placenta is not only the site of transport of nutrients from the cow's circulatory system to the foetus but it also plays an important role in the removal of waste products from the foetal circulatory system as well as the hormonal control of maintainance of pregnancy. Endocrine secretions (hormones and growth factors) from the placenta also help to maintain the growth and development of the calf. The transfer of nutrients across the placenta is controlled by a number of factors, the degree of apposition of the placenta to the endometrium (the surface area of the placenta), the rate of blood flow in the uterus and the umbilical cord and the efficiency of each of the individual nutrient transfer processes.

The main substances that are transported across the placenta are respiratory gases, glucose, lactic acid, lipids, amino acids and proteins, water, minerals, electrolytes and vitamins. The transfer of nutrients across the placenta occurs by one of four basic processes;

1. Simple diffusion (for example respiratory gases)

2. Facilitated diffusion (for example glucose)
3. Active transport - an energy requiring process (for example amino acids)
4. Pinocytosis - engulfment of a molecule in a lipid membrane and then transfer from one cell type to the next (for example proteins).

2.3.3.1 Respiratory gases: oxygen and carbon dioxide

The uterus and the placenta (not including the foetus) account for less than 20% of the weight of the pregnant (gravid) uterus in late pregnancy, but they use about 35 to 50% of all oxygen supplied. This highlights the intense metabolic processes in the uterus and placenta that are essential for maintaining the growing calf. Oxygen is passed from the maternal blood to the foetal blood by simple diffusion. In theory the transfer of oxygen to the foetus should be 100% efficient but various factors reduce the efficiency. One of the most important factors reducing the efficiency of oxygen transfer is the difference in the binding of oxygen to the cow's haemoglobin and the foetal haemoglobin. Other factors are the effect of apposition of the placenta to the endometrium (that is where and how frequently the two circulation systems meet), the rate of flow of blood to the uterus, the flow in the umbilical cord and the clearance of carbon dioxide by the placenta. The stage of pregnancy also plays an important role in the efficiency of transfer of oxygen. In many species immediately before parturition, a reduction in transfer is observed as there is an increase in uterine blood flow as a result of the increased physical activity of the uterine wall.

The intense metabolic activity of the placenta and the developing calf leads to the formation of high concentrations of carbon dioxide. The clearance of carbon dioxide occurs by diffusion. Again the diffusion should be 100% efficient but, the majority of carbon dioxide is carried in the blood as bicarbonate in fact. Very little bicarbonate is transferred directly from the foetus via the placenta to the maternal blood supply as there is little difference in concentration between the cow and the calf. The placental membrane appears to have also has a low permeability to bicarbonate. The majority of carbon dioxide produced by the foetus is transferred to the maternal blood system in a gaseous state. The placenta facilitates the conversion of carbon dioxide to bicarbonate by the enzyme carbonic anhydrase. The conversion allows the maternal blood to take up the carbon dioxide and carry it to the lungs for respiratory exchange.

2.3.3.2 Glucose and lactic acid

At least two thirds of the glucose taken up by the pregnant uterus is utilised by the placenta. The main reason for this high use of glucose in the placenta is the high demand of the foetus for amino acids. Amino acid transfer is an energy demanding process and therefore the supply of glucose and other energy yielding compounds must be maintained to ensure normal foetal growth. The majority of the glucose is converted to carbon dioxide but about 35% is converted to lactic acid and released to both the cow and the foetus.

Glucose is transported to the foetus from the cow by the process of facilitative diffusion. Specialised proteins in the placental membranes allow the glucose molecules to pass across the membrane of the maternal blood system to the foetal circulatory system. As the concentration of glucose in the cow's blood is greater than the foetal blood, transfer occurs at no cost of energy. The transport is however controlled by maintaining a relatively fixed ratio of concentrations between the cow and the calf. In periods of malnutrition in late pregnancy, the supply of glucose may be restricted to the calf if the concentration in the cow's blood declines. This may lead to dysfunction of the placenta and potentially reduced foetal growth. It is usually unlikely that the supply of glucose will be reduced to such an extent that significant damage to the foetus occurs. However, the ultimate size of foetus may be slightly smaller than if nutrition had been normal.

Lactic acid formation, as a result of use of glucose in conditions of low oxygen concentrations, can occur relatively rapidly in the placenta. It is the second most important source of carbohydrate supplied to the developing calf.

2.3.3.3 Fats (lipids)

The transfer across the ruminant placenta of short and long-chain fatty acids and ketones (3- hydroxy butyrate) is limited. Lipids cannot cross the placenta in an un-modified form. The fatty acids have to be converted to free fatty acids (for example acetate) and glycerol in the placenta. The use of glucose and lactic acid by the calf amounts to about 50% of its requirement for energy for growth. The free fatty acid acetate is exceptionally important in late pregnancy supplying about 15% of the energy requirement of the growing calf. The majority of ruminants are born with low reserves of body fat and they tend to have placenta which has a lower permeability to lipid than other species whose young have high levels of fat stored at birth (e.g. monkeys and humans). During pregnancy, the pregnant uterus also has a requirement for acetate and 3-hydroxybutyrate (a ketone) but it is unlikely that these compounds are used by the foetus for growth.

2.3.3.4 Amino acids and proteins

Only about 60 to 70% of the energy requirement of the calf has been accounted for by glucose, lactic acid or acetate. Amino acids have therefore an important role in foetal energy metabolism. This observation was made when it was noted that only about 50% of the amino acids which had been transfered to the calf were deposited into protein. This may seem unusual but it has been recognised that the breakdown of amino acids can yield a substantial amount of energy for metabolism. In late pregnancy the requirement of the developing calf for amino acids used as an energy source may be three times that required for tissue deposition.

The placenta also requires a supply of amino acids to ensure its own function. The bovine placenta continues to grow until about 230 days of pregnancy. The rate of amino acid incorporation into the placenta is however relative low (about 7 g per day). Measurements have been made to determine the net requirement of amino acids in the placenta and have shown the rate of use of amino acids is greater than the deposition of protein. There must be another role for amino acids in the placenta but it has not been fully researched.

Proteins are large molecules and therefore the transfer of the molecule across the placenta is difficult. Proteins are generally transferred across the placenta by a process known as pinocytosis (engulfment of the protein in a lipid membrane and then transfer to another cell). The most important proteins to be transferred from the cow to the calf are immunoglobins. The highest uptake of immunoglobulins by the calf is after parturition. These confer a degree of protection from infection to the developing calf which is maintained throughout the early stages of growth after birth. During periods of malnutrition in pregnancy, the impact of a reduction in the intake of protein by the cow is very small. Unlike glucose and other energy yielding substances, the concentration of amino acids in the cow's blood is reduced but there is not the concurrent reduction in amino acid concentration in the foetal blood. It is therefore a sensible strategy by the calf to utilise amino acids as an energy source. The constant removal of amino acids from the cow's blood by the foetus may pose a problem to her in the short term but mobilisation of body reserves during periods of poor nutrition allows the transfer and supply of amino acids to the calf to be maintained.

2.3.3.5 Water and electrolytes

Water is essential for all life and it is a "true" nutrient. There is a linear relationship between foetal wet and dry weight and uterine wet and dry weight, even during the last three months of pregnancy when most of the foetal body weight is accumulated. This would suggest there is an equal influx and efflux of water from the pregnant uterus during the whole of the pregnancy. The majority of water gained by the developing calf is derived from the cow's blood system. Some water is generated as a result of the breakdown of glucose, lactic acid and amino acids, however it is not known how much these supplies affect the uptake of water from the cow's blood. Water must pass from the cow to the foetus by the process of simple diffusion, a process which is likely to be regulated by the overall electrolyte balance across the placenta. The maintenance of the influx and efflux of water by the pregnant uterus is very important to ensure the amniotic fluid (the fluid that surrounds the calf) is maintained in an isotonic state compared to the calf and the placenta (that is a similar concentration of electrolytes in the water associated with amniotic fluid, calf and placenta). Amniotic fluid is swallowed by the calf throughout pregnancy and in sheep it has been estimated that about 30% of fluid swallowed is taken up by the gut and passed to the foetal blood.

Electrolytes (sodium, potassium, calcium, magnesium, chloride, sulphate and phosphate) are integral components of the blood plasma. They confer the stability to certain proteins in the blood (especially albumin), play an important role in the function of red blood cells and help to keep blood pressure stable. In general the concentrations of the individual electrolytes are higher in foetal blood than that of the cow's blood. This may pose a problem to regulation of transfer of nutrients across the placenta, for instance how does the placenta prevent a massive influx of water into the calf from the cow's circulatory system? The fetomaternal barrier is highly selective in its processes and therefore the complex regulation of transfer of electrolytes to and from the calf prevents massive flows of nutrients in either direction.

Uptake of amino acids by the placenta and the developing calf requires energy to drive the active transfer from the mother to the calf. This active transport requires the presence of sodium. The foetus can supply sodium to ensure the amino acid transfer occurs across the fetomaternal barrier and the cow's blood replaces the sodium by diffusion to the calf.

The rates of accretion of sodium, potassium, magnesium and chloride are generally linear throughout pregnancy. This would suggest that these electrolytes control the flow of water to and from the calf and the mother. It seems rather surprising that the accretion of sodium increases linearly throughout pregnancy as the amino acid requirement of the developing calf increases exponentially during the last five months of pregnancy. Only calcium and phosphate show an exponential increase in accumulation in the developing calf as pregnancy advances. This reflects the increase in the rate of mineralisation of bones in the calf with the greatest increases in rate of accumulation occurring in the last three months of pregnancy.

2.3.3.6 Trace elements

Little is known about the mechanisms of transfer of many of the trace elements across the placenta. The rate of accumulation of copper, zinc, manganese and iron into the developing calf corresponds directly to the stage of pregnancy and correlates strongly with total uterine uptake. The uptakes of iron and zinc are approximately ten times greater than of copper and manganese.

Iron is essential for the formation of haemoglobin, myoglobin and ferritin (an iron rich protein that acts as a temporary store for iron). Iron uptake by the foetus seems to be a two stage process. In stage one, an iron rich protein (transferritin) in the blood binds to special receptor sites in the placenta whereupon the iron is released from the protein. Stage two occurs when the free iron is either tranferred directly to the foetus or is re-stored for future use in the placenta in ferritin (compartmentation of iron in the placenta).

The concentration of free zinc in the blood is very low as the majority of the element is associated with protein (albumin). Zinc is essential for the normal development of the calf as it plays an important role in red blood cell formation, nucleic acid metabolism, protein synthesis and energy utilisation. The concentration of zinc is generally greater in the foetal blood and therefore to ensure zinc is transported across the placenta from the cow's blood to the foetus, it is closely associated with the transfer of amino acids or proteins.

2.3.3.7 Vitamins

The concentrations of water soluble vitamins (B, C, folate and biotin) in the blood of the cow are nearly always greater than the concentrations in the foetal blood. The converse is observed with fat soluble vitamins (A, D, E and K). The supply of these fat soluble vitamins to the calf is crucial for the correct development of the calf. The method of transport of fat soluble vitamins across the placenta occurs in association with specialised "carrier" proteins. Most water soluble vitamins cross the placenta by, presumably, the process of simple diffusion, but vitamin B12 and folate have to be transported by "carrier" protein systems.

2.4 Foetal growth

The requirement of the pregnant uterus for nutrients reflects the rate of growth of the placenta, the maintenance of the uterus itself and the growth of the developing calf. As previously mentioned, unlike sheep, the bovine placenta is still growing in the last part of pregnancy (after 230 days), albeit at a reduced rate. The pattern of growth of the placenta is very difficult to monitor as its structure (a cotyledon-type placenta) is highly complex and hence the full true requirement of it for energy, protein and other nutrients have not been elucidated. This poses a theoretical problem for rationing the animal during late pregnancy.

Over the whole pregnancy, the growth of the foetus is exponential by time from conception. More than 60% of the total birth-weight of the calf is deposited during the last two months of pregnancy. Therefore, the maximum requirement for nutrients occurs during the dry period. In a detailed study in the United States using Holstein cows, foetal growth between day 190 and 270 showed the average rate of growth of the calf was 418 g/day (or 121 g DM/day) with no tail off in growth after 230 days of pregnancy. In previous studies, declines in the rate of growth of the calf were observed after 230 days of pregnancy. This decline in rate of growth was thought to reflect a reduction in the efficiency of the placenta (hyperplasia or hypertrophy of the placenta). The finding that there was little if any reduction in the rate of growth of the calf during late pregnancy is even more important as an acknowledgement of continuing growth to the last week of pregnancy must lead to the conclusion that the cow must be fed correctly to term.

During pregnancy the cow must facilitate storage of fat, protein, mineral matter in the developing calf. In a 40 kg calf (at 40 weeks term) approximately 73% of body weight is water, 3.5% is fat and 19% is protein. Mineral matter (bone, teeth and minerals associated with body fluids and tissue makes up the other 4.5% of body weight. As mentioned previously, over 60% of the projected birth-weight of the calf is deposited in the last eight weeks of pregnancy - the dry period.

The weight of fat, protein and mineral matter deposited in the amniotic fluid, membranes and the pregnant uterus is relatively low compared to the contribution of nutrients to the calf. The cow must deposit nutrients in the amniotic fluid (about a 50:50 ratio of protein and mineral matter in the dry matter of the fluid), foetal membranes (mainly protein and lipid) and the uterus (about 80% of the deposition is protein) during pregnancy the cow must facilitate enough nutrients to allow the deposition of each component. The levels of fat, protein and mineral matter deposited in the calf and the pregnant uterus at term are 1.6, 9.6and 2.6 kg respectively. If she does not allow this transfer, there may be the risk of a non-viable calf.

2.4.1 Nutrient prioritisation

Foetal growth is determined and prioritised by the flow of nutrients from the cow to the calf across the placenta as well as by genetic and maternal factors. It should be stressed that the priority of the cow is to maintain her own body systems (requirements for maintenance and growth in the heifer) and not to sustain pregnancy at all costs.

The detailed requirements of the foetus for various nutrients were discussed in the previous sections but no information was presented on how to quantify the requirements nor the relative demands on the cow's own body reserves. This section considers the supply of nutrients to the foetus in relation to the priorities set by the cow.

The priority of nutrients supply to the foetus is as follows :

Nutrient	**Priority to foetus**
Oxygen	High
Energy substrates (glucose, lactic acid, amino acids)	High
Tissue construction (amino acids)	High
Insulin (carbohydrate and energy control)	High
Growth factors (IGF)	High
Energy substrates (lipids)	Moderate
Thyroid, growth hormones and cortisol	Moderate

Nutrients released from feeds by fermentative and digestive processes enter intermediary metabolism as the raw materials to be partitioned to sites of requirement. Nutrients are partitioned to all body tissues that support productive function (mammary gland, muscles, liver, gastro-intestinal tract and reproductive tract). This process is the result of the homeorhetic regulation of metabolism rather than an equal division of nutrients to all sites of need. The order of priority set by the cow is suggested as the maintenance of her own body tissues, pregnancy, growth (if occurring), lactation, deposition of reserves (fat and protein) and the ability to reproduce (ovarian activity and reproductive cyclicity).

In the heifer, growth may well be a greater priority to pregnancy. One of the best practical examples cited to describe this effect is the prioritisation of nutrients in the growing heifer. If the animal has been served at too young an age or is of too small frame size, the level of feed allowance may be reduced to try to ensure the calf is of a small size. The effect of lowering feed allowance is to reduce the growth rate of the heifer rather than reduce the rate of growth of the calf. The risk of dystocia may well be increased as a disproportionately large calf to the size of the heifer will be produced.

The energy requirement of the foetus has to be met mainly by the supply of glucose. The rate of transfer of glucose from the cow's circulation to the developing calf is dependent on the relative concentration of glucose on either side of the placenta barrier. The incidence of hypoglycaemia (low concentrations in glucose in the blood) in late pregnancy may reduce the supply of glucose to the foetus. The increased demand for glucose in very late pregnancy may not be sustained without a change in type of ration. If changes are not made in the ration in late pregnancy, or are made too late, the incidence of hypoglycaemia in late pregnancy may well be increased. It is also important to note that the efficiency of utilisation of metabolisable energy of the conceptus is the lowest (0.133) of all the efficiencies of utilisation (for more details see Chapter 5).

How does the foetus cope with any fluctuations in and the changes in supply of glucose? Any decline in the concentration of glucose in the cow's blood and thus the supply to the foetus can be dealt with efficiently by an increase in the utilisation of amino acids as the energy substrate. This use of amino acids to yield energy is at the expense of protein synthesis in the calf and therefore a depression in the rate of growth of the foetus. The depression in foetal growth is observed by an increase in the output of ammonia and urea (waste by-products of amino acid breakdown) by the placenta. The under-supply of glucose to the foetus is likely to be transient as the response of the cow is rapid to rectify the problem.

The regulation of energy supply is controlled by insulin, growth hormone (bovine somaotrophin, bST) and cortisol. The role of maternal hormonal control on foetal growth is related to nutritional regulation rather than direct regulation of growth of foetus. Hormones from the cow do not cross the placenta in high enough concentrations to affect the growth and development of the calf and therefore the regulation of nutrients and the control of the processes of partition of nutrients received by the foetus is performed by the foetus itself. If the cow detects a reduction in glucose in its circulation, it increases the concentration of circulatory non-esterified fatty acids (NEFA) and ketones.

The NEFA and ketones are converted in the liver and the supply of glucose to the developing calf is increased and maintained at normal concentrations. Partial or complete breakdown of NEFA leads to an increase in the concentration of 3-hydroxybutyrate. This compound can be used by the pregnant uterus as an energy source thus ensuring the level of energy is not reduced. Increases in the concentration of NEFA and ketones occur in late pregnancy even under normal feeding regimes. These increases may well be under strict control by the changes in the endocrine status of the cow. During days 260 to 280 of pregnancy, the concentration of NEFA increases rapidly even in well-fed cattle. Does the increase in NEFA reflect the increases in the oestrogen:progesterone ratio or reflect a decline in voluntary intake of nutrients? The answer at present is not known, but increasing the intake of energy immediately before calving does not affect the change in NEFA concentration. Maybe the increase is related to the onset of the calving process where rapidly available energy supplies to muscle and uterine metabolism are required. If underfeeding occurs during late pregnancy, it is likely that the increased concentrations of NEFA and ketones in the blood are compounded by the natural rise in concentration thus increasing the risk of ketosis immediately after calving.

When over-feeding of energy takes place during the dry period, the cow increases the risk of impairing liver function in early lactation. Lipid mobilisation is a normal physiological process in early lactation ("milking-off her back"), but if the cow carries excessive condition the metabolic disorder of fatty liver may occur. As a consequence the output of energy substrates from the liver in early lactation is markedly reduced as there is an increase in the mobilisation of fat from adipose tissue stores. For a more detailed discussion of the effect of excessive condition in late pregnancy see Chapter 6.

Further recommended reading

Battaglia, F.C. and Meschia, G. (1986) *An Introduction to Fetal Physiology*. Academic Press, New York.

Bell, A.W. (1993) Pregnancy and Fetal Metabolism. 405-431. In, J.M. Forbes and J. France (eds). *Quantitative Aspects of Ruminant Digestion and Metabolism*. CAB International, Wallingford, UK.

Bell, A.W. (1995) Regulation of organic nutrient metabolism during transition from late pregnancy to early lactation. *Journal of Animal Science* **73**: 2804.

Bell, A.W., Slepetis, R. and Ehrhardt, R.A. (1995) Growth and accretion of energy and protein in the gravid uterus during late pregnancy in Holstein cows. *Journal of Dairy Science* **78**: 1954.

Davis, C.L. and Drackley, J.K. (1998) *The Development, Nutrition and Management of the Young Calf.* Iowa State University Press, Ames, USA.

Ginther, O.J. (1998) *Ultrasonic Imaging and Animal Reproduction: Cattle.* EquiService Publishing, USA.

Grummer, R.R. (1995) Impact of changes in organic nutrient metabolism on feeding the transition dairy cow. *Journal of Animal Science* **73**: 2820.

Longo, L.D. and Reneau, D.D. (1978) *Fetal and Newborn Cardiovascular Physiology.* Raven Press, New York.

Peters, A.R. and Ball, P.J.H. (1995) *Reproduction in Cattle.* Blackwell Science, Oxford, UK.

Peters, A.R. and Ball, P.J.H. (1999) Priorities for research and technology transfer for the improvement of dairy cattle reproduction. *Milk Development Council Report,* 1999.

Roberts, R.M. (1989) Conceptus interferons and maternal recognition of pregnancy. *Biology of Reproduction,* **40**: 449.

Roy, J.H.B. (1980) *The Calf, Fourth Edition.* Butterworths, London, UK.

Wassell, T.R. and Esslemont, R.J. (1992) Herd Health Schemes; their scope and use by dairy farmers. *Farm Management* **8**: 194.

Chapter 3

DRY COW MANAGEMENT

This chapter concentrates on the methods that can be applied when drying off cows, the implications of drying off cows abruptly or not on udder development and function, the duration of the dry period, dry cow therapy and the control of various diseases of the udder that may occur during the dry period, for instance summer mastitis.

3.1 Factors influencing udder development

Udder development is very important to successful milk production. The gland basically consists of parenchymal tissue which contains the alveoli (secretory tissue) where milk is produced. The growth of the mammary gland (udder) follows a two-stage developmental pattern. The first phase of rapid development occurs before the first pregnancy and is centred around puberty. The second phase (or many phases) is extensive growth and involution during successive cycles of pregnancy, lactation and dry periods.

During the initial post-natal period of mammary gland growth, the rate of growth is isometric compared to the relative growth rate of the cow. This means that the gland deposits tissue at a similar rate to that of the body carcase. To four months of age, a high plane of nutrition does not seem to effect the structural development of the mammary gland, but it may increase the size of the fat pad. This increase in fat pad size at an early stage of development may be important in the subsequent stages of development of the mammary gland. However, during the period 3 to 6 months of age, there is an increase in the rate of mammary gland growth. This elevated rate of deposition of tissue continues until about 2 to 3 months after the first oestrous. Until pregnancy, the tissue deposition of the developing mammary gland is characterised by double-layered, densely packed ductular epithelium and supporting stromal cells which grow into the fat pad. The size of the fat pad varies according to energy intake and if energy consumption is high during the pre-pubertal phase, there is an associated reduction in growth of parenchyma. This can result in a switch in the partitioning of nutrients and lead to carcase fattening and/or fat deposition in the mammary gland, which may lead to a reduction in future lactational performance. It is therefore essential that calves, even at this early stage of development are monitored for rapid changes in condition. After puberty, a high plane of nutrition and fat deposition have not been associated with detrimental effects on parenchymal growth and therefore have little effect on subsequent milk production.

Alveolar proliferation is regulated by the hormones progesterone and prolactin. While placental lactogen (a hormone produced by the placenta that has a role in "switching-on" lactation in mammals) may stimulate alveolar development and proliferation in some species, this is not the case in cattle as little hormone enters the maternal blood circulation. Limited cell proliferation occurs after calving and the majority of the increase in yield of milk during early lactation can be ascribed to an increase activity per cell to produce milk. During late lactation and the dry period, the reverse applies when falling yield of milk leads to a reduction in cell activity and an acceleration in potentially cell loss. The duct system which transfers the milk from its site of production to the milk cistern and then out via the teat is complex and its development is important in ensuring maximum efficiency of the mammary gland during lactation. The duct system ranges from fine ducts that drain alveolar space and carry milk directly to the nipple to large galactophores which end as cisterns (elastic sinuses). Oestrogens and bovine somatotropin (bST) are responsible for duct formation. The presence of corticosteroids, produced by the adrenal gland, helps to maximise the growth of the mammary gland.

In the heifer, a high plane of nutrition results in rapid body weight and condition score increased in heifers between 100 and 300 kg, and tends to reduce the weight of the mammary gland secretory tissue thus reducing subsequent milk production. In many such instances there is excessive fat deposited in the udder. The main reason for this observation is probably a reduction in bovine somatotropin production. It appears that an injection of bST increases parenchymal development and so it might be possible to re-partition nutrients in the well-fed animal to ensure mammary and other tissue development rather than fat deposition. It is clear that the management of the heifer prior to puberty influences the productive capability of the mature cow and therefore careful control of her nutrition reduces the incidence of animals with reduced lactational performance.

Finally, it is important to observe the following rules. Condition scoring of cattle during the pre-pubertal to puberty phase of growth is essential for all elite animals. If inadequate monitoring of condition score occurs and the animal starts to deposit fat in her carcase rapidly, there will be a reduction in potential milk yield. Some nutritionists advocate the rule that growth of the maiden heifer must not exceed her final predicted weight in grammes per day. Therefore if the predicted weight of the cow is to be 650 kg, the heifer should not grow at a rate of greater than 650 g/day.

3.2 Duration of the dry period

Throughout lactation, udder development continues and there is constant repair and synthesis of udder parenchymal tissues. Udder development is reversed in advanced lactation when gradual involution occurs. This effect is even more pronounced in the dry period. A period of non-production is essential for maximum milk production in the next lactation. Yield of milk in the next lactation is impaired if the dry period is less than six weeks. However, there appears to be little advantage in extending the dry period longer than eight weeks in average cows. Overfeeding in late lactation and in the dry period may have a similar effect to that in the growing heifer in reducing the regeneration of milk secretory tissue.

After drying off, the mammary gland gradually changes. There is an initial period when milk secretion builds up, thus excreting an increased internal pressure on the milk secretory tissues and preventing further production. This suppression of milk synthesis will continue unless milk is drawn off. Usually the suppression will only be broken if milk is drawn off by the milker (a procedure in once a day milking systems) or the cow is otherwise so stimulated that she lets down her milk and she leaks milk. Fluid pressure within the udder increases for the first few days but usually starts to decrease after the third day. However it takes until the sixth day or longer before the pressure in the udder is the same or less than that occurring at 12 hours after milking during her lactation.

Following the reduction in udder pressure and during the next 30 days, the mammary gland undergoes a period of involution. This involves the active absorption of components of the milk secretory tissue into the animal's body system. There is then a quiescent phase that will vary depending on the time left before calving. This is followed by a period lasting 15 to 20 days when there is active formation of colostrum and milk (the lactogenic period). Thus as the involution phase takes about 30 days and the lactogenic period 15 to 20 days it does mean that the dry period needs to be at least 45 to 50 days long (about six to seven weeks).

3.3 Drying off

It is best to dry cows off abruptly. This is achieved by stopping milking completely. The cow should be removed from a high energy diet and either have a reduced quantity or quality of feed. Some farmers advocate drying the cow off slowly by milking once a day. However, if this is done all the wrong stimuli are being given to the cow who, in consequence, will be activated into continued milk production. Also the extended period between milkings allows any infections which enter the udder a longer period to become established. While only being milked once a day, if she is kept with the main herd she will be stimulated by being collected with the others for milking even if she does not go through the parlour. This may well cause her to eject milk from her teats. If she is milking she will continue to be fed for the milk which she is producing and this again promotes milk production. If she is not fed adequately and is still actively yielding a quantity of milk she will then start to lose condition. This may have a detrimental effect in the next lactation and also influence the development of ova that will be used for producing the next calf during the forthcoming lactation. The mechanism of restriction of milk synthesis is related to the production of an inhibitory protein which acts in the mammary synthetic tissue. If the inhibitor is removed frequently (that is the cow is milked) the rate of milk secretion is high. However, reduce the rate of removal of the inhibitor protein (stop milking the cow) and a reduction in milk synthesis occurs.

It is essential that infusion of dry cow intra-mammary tubes (dry cow therapy) is undertaken in an absolutely clean environment. Obviously any infection that enters the teats has a period of several weeks to reside in the udder rather than the period between milkings that occurs in the lactating cow. The cowman should wear gloves when inserting the dry cow tubes and clean his hands in disinfectant water between cows or more frequently if they become contaminated. This should be done after the last milking and the cows should be treated in a clean place such as the parlour after milking has finished and the parlour has been washed down and is clean. The parlour is ideal as the teats are at the right height for ensuring effective infusion.

The cows should have the ends of the teats cleaned with a disposable swab soaked in spirit and then the tube inserted. The teats should then be dipped. The milker should infuse the teats furthest away from him first and then those closest to him. The teat dipping should be in the reverse order to the insertion to try and reduce contamination. Infusion should not be undertaken in a collecting yard or in a crush unless it is impossible to do it in the parlour. If a crush or collecting yard is used they again have to be thoroughly cleaned before the cows enter. If foot timing is going to be done, this should not take place at the same time. Cows should be kept somewhere close by, so that their udders can be watched in the next few days after drying off.

During the dry period, the udders and teats should be inspected frequently and in the summer ideally twice daily. The udder secretions should not be expressed unless it is thought there is something abnormal present. Teat dipping should be practised as an aid to keeping teats clean and reduce surface bacteria and to indirectly to allow enforced examination of the cow and her udder. It is particularly beneficial in the last ten days or so before calving. At this time the udder is again becoming susceptible to new infections including those of summer mastitis and the antibiotic in the dry cow therapy may be reduced in concentration or, if the dry period is long, no longer present

If dry cow therapy is used, and gradual drying off is adopted, then there is the problem as to when to use the intramammary tube. They obviously cannot be used while the cow is still milking. In once a day systems the increased length between milkings allows more time for any bacteria entering the udder to multiply and so cause immediate disease or remain in the udder to produce problems later. There is no problem in abruptly drying off a cow even when producing 30 litres of milk. All that is necessary is to stop milking, insert dry cow therapy and keep the cow on a diet of straw or poor quality hay for a few days (usually three or four days will suffice). If she were kept on a production ration, she would be stimulated to produce milk and so would develop a very swollen, udder and show discomfort. It is necessary to ensure adequate access to water for the cow at all times during the drying off period.

3.4 Infections of the udder in the dry period

The dry period is a time when new infections can enter the udder. Much can be done to prevent this from happening and also the removal of infections already present can be achieved. If cows are housed inside during the dry period and the conditions of housing are not kept clean then there is likely to be much exposure to environmental pathogens and as calving approaches and occurs, the risk of environmental mastitis becomes very high. Even outside, cows have to be kept very tightly stocked to prevent an increase in condition score and milk fever. Such areas will often have a very high level of bacterial contamination that can be just as bad as for animals kept inside. This can become a particularly severe problem if summer conditions at pasture are poor (wet, muddy conditions). In the summer there is also the added danger of summer mastitis.

3.4.1 Treatment of infections already present in the udder

Staphylococcus aureus The treatment of *Staphylococcus aureus* infections in the lactating cow is difficult and often unsuccessful. This is despite the bacteria usually being sensitive to a range of antibiotics in the laboratory tests. The problem is mainly because *S. aureus* takes refuge in the white cells in the blood (polymorphonuclear neutrophils and macrophages where they are found in the cells). Most antibiotics diffuse poorly into these white cells and even if they enter the cells they may not pass into the phagolysosomes. Thus successful treatment in lactation depends on more prolonged courses of antibiotics than those usually recommended and such action will obviously involve a long period of milk withdrawal from sale. Obviously long therapeutic antibiotic activity is much more easily obtainable when there are no milk withhold worries.

Streptococcus uberis While infection can be present in the udder, it can also be found in the tonsils, gut, reproductive tract and the environment. It is therefore impossible to eradicate the pathogen. The infection can also be present in the udder at drying off, but equally it can enter during the dry period. *Streptococcus uberis* can also be found in cases of summer mastitis. Thus control of the infection does depend on maintaining high concentrations of suitable antibiotics in the udder throughout the dry period.

Streptococcus dysgalactiae This organism can reside in the udder, but it is also found outside it. Infections can be present in the udder at drying off and, on occasions, they can also be contracted during the dry period. The organism is usually susceptible to a range of antibiotics (for example penicillin, eythromycin, cloxacillin and the cephalosporins).

Streptococcus agalactiae This organism can only survive in the udder except for short periods on the skin of the cow or the cowman. It was once the most common cause of mastitis, however herds which have diligently practised effective treatment of clinical cases, used post milking dipping and dry cow therapy have usually eliminated the problem. However, the infection is still often seen in herds illustrating that the control of mastitis could be improved. The organism can be well regulated by dry cow therapy and it is usually sensitive to the same antibiotics as *Streptococcus dysgalatiae.*

3.4.2 Prevention of new infections entering the udder during the dry period

It has been shown that dry cow therapy preparations that have an extended duration of activity (that is longer than the traditional three to four weeks) reduce the number of pathogenic bacteria that can be isolated at the subsequent calving. New infections of several pathogens can occur during the dry period.

Escherichia coli The udder of the dry cow generally possesses natural resistance to infection with *Escherichia coli.* The main reason for this is that *E. coli* and other gram-negative bacteria require iron to multiply. However, during the dry period almost all the available iron present in the mammary gland is taken up in the formation of lactoferrin (an iron rich protein) and so is unavailable for bacterial use, thereby inhibiting their growth and establishment. Alteration of this situation does not occur until a few days before calving.

Streptococcus uberis While infection of this organism can come from the previous lactation the dry period is often a major time when new infections are contracted. It is the most common new infection of the dry period, with most invasion occurring in the first or last two weeks of the period. Provided an appropriate antibiotic is used in the dry period, infections in the early period (first two weeks after drying off) will be killed off. However, those infections occurring in the last two weeks of the dry period may well not be removed and therefore can cause a problem in the subsequent lactation.

Streptococcus dysgalatiae This pathogen is less contagious than other *Streptococcus* infections (such as *Streptococcus agalatiae*), but new infections can occur at this time.

Arcanobacterium pyogenes Summer mastitis is a very common problem in the dry cow during the summer months. While several organisms can be involved in this problem *Arcanobacterium* (formerly *Actinomyces*; formerly *Corynebacterium*) *pyogenes* is usually accepted to be the most important. This organism gains entry in the dry period and so, if prevention is required, it is necessary for the dry cow therapy to contain the appropriate antibiotic. some suitable antibiotics include cloxacillin, nafcillin and the cephalosporins. If the dry period is likely to be long and there is the possibility that summer mastitis might occur, it is often better to use an effective antibiotic in a preparation with an extended duration of activity. This allows protection to be provided without the need to repeat treatment. Several other organisms can be found on their own or in mixed infections often with *Arcanobacterium pyogenes*. The one reported to produce the characteristic smell of summer mastitis is known as *Peptococcus indolicus.*

3.4.3 Duration of dry cow therapy

Dry cow therapy has two main purposes:

1. To treat infections already present in the udder and,
2. To prevent entry of new infections during the dry period.

Dry cow therapy depends on the prolonged release of antibiotic over a considerable period of time. This can be achieved by several methods including the adjustment of particle size, the addition of slow release bases such as certain vegetable and mineral oils, aluminium monostearate and the use of insoluble salts such as the benzathine form of penicillin. In some instances the oil method provides an extension of activity by providing the antibiotic in a hydrophobic vehicle.

In the past, most antibiotics used in the dry cow had a duration of activity of about three to four weeks. This meant that if the dry period was longer then the udder would not be protected from attack by pathogenic organisms. New infections could become established and result in disease in the second half of the dry period or at calving. This leads to the dilemma as to whether a second dose of antibiotic should be given. If this second tube insertion was not done the cow would be vulnerable to disease. However, if done, the teat seal was broken and if done badly or by an unhygienic method, damage could be done to the teat or infection introduced. Another problem was that if the cow only had another two weeks or so before she calved then there was a chance that she would give birth before the activity of the antibiotic had finished and so several days of early milk production would be unable to be sold. This now has been virtually eliminated by the introduction of dry cow tubes with extended periods of activity ranging from seven to ten weeks. In some instances the choice of dry cow tube will as much depend on the expected dry period as on the antibiotic present within it. Where dry periods are likely to vary, it is best to work out a range of preparations for those with a short, normal (six weeks) or extended dry period.

3.5 The early calving cow

When a cow calves early and so the dry cow therapy antibiotic may still be persistent in the udder, there are two possible courses of action. Firstly to withhold the milk from the bulk tank for the minimum time of treatment. This is usually the time to elapse for duration of activity in the udder plus the minimum time from calving until the milk can be offered for human consumption. This period however will need to be altered depending on any contractual obligations with the milk purchaser. Otherwise it is possible to test the milk for antibiotic residues routinely until it is clear. This may be of particular benefit if the period of milk wastage is likely to be prolonged. The testing should be undertaken by a reputable laboratory.

Due to commercial interests of milk buyers, reliable data are not available on milk antibiotic failures or their cause. However in the mid 1980s, early calving or short dry periods resulted in 6.6% of failures (1983/4) and 7.3% (1984/5). Accidental milking of dry cows resulted in 5.1% and 6.2% failure for the same periods respectively. Use of a dry cow preparation during lactation also resulted in 0.9% and 0.8% of all problems in those years. It is essential that accurate records are kept of cows treated with dry cow therapy and when their milk is safe to enter the bulk tank. All intramammary tubes must be used according to the number and interval between tube insertion according to the manufacturers data sheets. If these instructions are not followed then a standard withdrawal time should be used which is seven days. Communication with staff is the key step to ensure that failure does not occur as a result of antibiotic treatment. In addition all freshly calved cows should be easily identifiable by all who milk the cows. Dry cow therapy should be kept in a different place from all other forms of treatment both intramammary tubes, injections and drenches.

While most antibiotic failures following use of dry cow therapy are the result of human error, a few cannot be ascribed to this cause. A few appear to be due to cows having an individually long udder persistence of the antibiotic. Thus some of these cows studied with such problems have had persistence times greater than twice the normal. In certain of these animals, cystic structures of variable size have been found in the mammary tissue often in the region of the milk cistern. Fluid in these structures can contain antibiotics.

The use of appropriate antibiotic injections has been advocated for assisting in the elimination of persistent mammary infections. Any antibiotics used must be able to enter and concentrate in the udder. The one most commonly used is tylosin. It has produced good results in some chronic mastitis problems, but it is not always successful.

3.6 Summer mastitis

Summer mastitis is almost always seen in the dry cow, heifer and even occasionally the bull. Invariably it is many times more common as calving approaches. It is generally thought to be caused by *Arcanobacterium (Actinomyces) pyogenes* often in conjunction with other organisms such as *Peptococcus indolicus* (a micrococcus) which is claimed to give the secretions their foul smell. Many other organisms can be isolated including microaerophilic cocci, *Streptococcus uberis* and *Streptococcus dysgalatiae.* The condition tends to be seen in the summer, hence its name, with most cases occurring during August (resulting in the term "August bag"), but with some in June, July and September. However cases can occasionally be seen at other times of the year. The head fly, *Hydrotoea irritans*, has been incriminated in helping the spread of infection in herds. The fly is generally found near woodlands and often close to water.

The disease is usually seen in a peracute or acute form. The first sign is an increase in fly activity around the teats of the cow and is usually missed. There then follows a marked rise in temperature of the animal with the cow often away from the rest of the herd. In many cases she will appear lame when moved. The cow will not be eating much, will usually appear dull and will have a raised temperature of 40 to 41°C (104 to 106°F). One or more of the quarters will be swollen, reddened, hot and painful. If the teat is drawn, it will contain a purulent foul smelling yellow usually watery secretion but, in some instances, blood stained. In some animals the hock or fetlock will be swollen. Provided treatment is prompt, the animal will survive, but the quarter is invariably lost. As the disease proceeds the affected quarter will lose its heat, become hardened and often lumpy. These lumps are abcesses and they can rupture and exude thick pus to the outside.

Treatment involves the veterinary surgeon and the use of appropriate antibiotics and anti-inflammatory agents. The udder may need to have the teat removed to allow the escape of pus or the abcesses in the udder may need to be lanced. The affected cow should be removed from the rest of the herd as she will be a source of infection and attraction for flies which may settle on her teats and then alight on another animal. Once one case has occurred, others may follow and so the animals should be examined even more frequently than before and it is suggested they are moved away from areas likely to be frequented by the head fly.

Prevention of the disease includes the use of dry cow therapy using an appropriate antibiotic and ensuring the duration of activity will extend the whole length of the dry period. The use of a course or one injection of an appropriate long acting antibiotic can be helpful. Some suitable antibiotics include cloxacillin, nafcillin and the cephalosporins. If the dry period is likely to be long and there is the possibility that summer mastitis might occur, it is often better to use an effective antibiotic in a preparation with an extended duration of activity. This allows protection to be provided without the need to repeat treatment.

All dry cows should be inspected frequently, ideally twice a day. There is much point in taking the cows through the milking parlour while dry so that the teats can be teat dipped and this ensures that the teats and udders will be indirectly examined. Each cow should be checked for any damage or sores on her teats. These should be immediately and effectively treated as they tend to attract flies. If dry cows do pass through the parlour it should ideally be done at a time following milking and when all the milking machinery is switched off thereby reducing the likelihood of milk let down and ejection.

The use of teat tape can act as a barrier to the head fly. The treatment of all the cows with an appropriate ectoparasiticide as a wash, spray or ear tag may give some protection against the head fly as do some fly repellents. Farmers relying on ectoparasiticidal ear tags have had variable success with them. If they are to be used, then one per ear will be required to provide sufficient ectoparasiticide at the udder. In months when cattle are particularly vulnerable, the cows should be kept well away from likely head fly habitats. In areas or farms where the condition is particularly bad, thought should be given to calving at a different time of year. Work is being undertaken on preparations to coat the teat end and act as a sealant to it. These are available in some countries and have given success on cows on some farms. In the normal dry period, two applications may be required.

While attention has recently been focused on the necessity of using antibiotic dry cow therapy, it is at present the only reliable and tested method of controlling existing infections within the udder or the prevention of new ones. When used on a herd basis, it should always be used following a study of the bacteria present in the cows of that farm and their antibiotic sensitivities. There may be some valid argument that dry cow therapy is unnecessary in cattle which have never suffered clinical mastitis or a high cell count or are dry in the winter months. However such a strategy needs to be fully evaluated in terms of its likely consequences. On organic farms routine dry cow therapy of all cows is not acceptable. However a dry cow tube can be used on individual animals if it is justified by their high milk cell count. Usually the milk withhold time will be increased and advice should be sought from the organic organisation of which the producer is a member.

Further recommended reading

Andrews, A.H. (1990) *Outline of Clinical Diagnosis in Cattle.* Wright, London, UK.

Blowey, R.W. and Edmondson, P. (1995) *Mastitis Control in Dairy Herds.* Farming Press, Ipswich, UK.

Bramley, A.J., Dodd, F.H., Mein, G.A. and Bramley, J.A. (1992) *Milking Machine and Lactation.* Insight Books, Burlington, USA.

Knight, C.H., Brown, J.R. and Dewhurst, R.J. (1995). Udder characteristics and relationship to efficiency of milk production. 79-85. In, T.L.J. Lawrence, F.J. Gordon and A.Carson (eds) Breeding and Feeding the High Genetic Merit Dairy Cow. *BSAS Occasional Publication 19*, Edinburgh, UK.

Mepham, T.B. (1987). *Physiology of Lactation.* Open University Press, Milton Keynes, UK.

Chapter 4

CALVING

4.1 Signs prior to calving

There are several signs of approaching calving (parturition). Usually the first indication is the udder starting to enlarge, becoming swollen and tense. If the teats are drawn there is thick yellow colostrum present as birth becomes more imminent. Later the vulva starts to enlarge and often swells and about one to two days before parturition, there is the passage of clear vaginal mucus which has formed the seal to the cervix of the uterus during pregnancy. While this indicates calving is imminent, it does not give any exact fix on the time. Another useful sign is a fall in rectal temperature which will vary in degree and its timing before calving. Perhaps the best sign of imminent calving is the relaxation of the pelvic ligaments. As relaxation occurs, the base of the tail starts to become more prominent and the surrounding muscles appear sunken. The relaxation usually becomes marked in the last 24 hours before calving and there is also some loss of the tone within the tail. These signs are often the most useful guide of calving occurring within the next day. There is often a change in behaviour, with the cow separating from the remainder of the herd and usually seeking out a corner or less exposed area in which to calve.

4.2 Stages of calving

A normal calving can be divided into three stages, each is of variable duration and under normal circumstances various changes will occur during each stage.

4.2.1 First stage

During the first stage the calf starts to adopt the position for delivery, the cervix of the uterus will relax and expand, the uterus will commence to contract and the outer birth bag (the allantochorion) will enter the dilated cervix. These events are very variable in their duration but often appear to take little time in the cow which has had several pregnancies (multiparous), but can take a considerable period of time in heifers. The usual duration of this stage is from about 1 to 24 hours (average 6 hours). In many multiparous cows much of this stage is missed by the observer as it is accompanied by minimal signs and so it is often very difficult to be certain as to when first stage labour began. As said previously the tail head is invariably and noticeably raised. The main signs of the first stage of labour are usually of increasing unease and restlessness, with the cow stopping eating, she may circle, often going down and rapidly rising again, paddling her feet and in some cases pawing at the ground and, if straw or other loose bedding is present throwing it over herself. There is often a trembling of the flank muscles and in some animals there will be occasional straining.

Internally the cervix will become softer and dilates so that it is eventually not possible to determine its presence. The outer water bag (allantochorion) gradually passes through the cervix and enters the vagina. This allantochorion may appear intact at the vulva as a blue/purplish semitransparent thick walled covering containing blood vessels. In other instances it will rupture within the cervix or vagina and release a quantity of clear yellowish fluid. The division between first and second stage labour is often not very clear-cut.

4.2.2 Second stage

In this stage the calf initially enclosed in the inner water bag (the amnion) is delivered and abdominal muscle contractions occur as well as uterine. The second stage of labour is relatively short and should not last longer than half to about three hours (average about 70 minutes). While most cattle lie down to give birth, they can equally be successful in completing a calving while standing. Often the calf is present at the vulva in a white sac (inner water bag, amnion) and the features of the calf may be visible through it. The amniotic sac ruptures in over 80% of cases during delivery and this rupture generally takes place at the vulva. It may, however, have taken place previously at the cervix and or within the uterus itself. Usually rupture of the amniotic sac will be accompanied by increased straining movements. The cow will often put tremendous effort into the straining with arched back, extended legs and she will often groan or bellow. Once the head is present at the vulva, delivery is usually rapid. The umbilical cord often remains intact after delivery and only ruptures as the calf starts to stand or the cow rises.

4.2.3 Third stage

In the third stage, the placenta is expelled and this normally occurs within the next 12 hours although it can be as long as 24 hours later (average is about 6 hours). This period may involve uterine contractions as well as some abdominal contractions.

4.3 Assistance at calving

Wherever possible it is best to allow the calving process to occur naturally and not to interfere unnecessarily. If there is a compulsion to investigate then it should only be to determine that the calf is in the normal position with head and front feet presented. Normally first stage labour will vary and there should be no real problems if it lasts ten hours. However at the end of first stage the cow starts to show visible abdominal straining and the cervix should then be open. If the straining in second stage has been violent for half an hour without apparent progress then an investigation may be necessary. However if the cow has been periodically straining for two hours, or the amnion is at the vulva for about the equivalent time, it may be the normal process of calving or it is possible that there are problems. Thus at this stage it is best for the stockperson or veterinary surgeon to investigate and ensure that everything is normal. If, on examination, the cervix is not open then veterinary assistance should be requested. If however, all appears well then it is probably best to leave and check again in half an hour. If after three hours nothing has happened and the cervix is open and straining has been frequent then it may be necessary to intervene and attempt to calve the cow. If there are any doubts about what is happening, the veterinary surgeon should be called. It is possible for the calf to survive for up to eight hours during second stage labour when it is correctly presented. However this will not always be the case.

The main signs to give cause for concern are as follows.

(1) Anything which appears to be abnormal either in timing, in signs shown by the cow or following examination of the vulva, vagina, uterus or calf.

(2) The first stage labour lasting 24 hours (it is suggested animals are checked after 10 to 12 hours in case of problems).

(3) The first stage labour lasting more than 10 to12 hours without some relaxation of the cervix.

(4) The first stage labour where the cervix starts to relax but this does not continue.

(5) If the cow adopts abnormal positioning during the first stage labour. She may look in distress, call excessively, stand with her legs splayed out away from her body or have a dipped back.

(6) Excessive straining for more than half an hour without any signs of progress.

(7) If there has been no appearance of the amnion or calf in the vagina after two hours of intermittent straining (if nothing is present at the vulva, this can only be determined by a vaginal examination).

(8) If the amniotic sac is present at the vulva for two hours and there is no progress.

(9) If on manual examination the head or legs of the calf feel relatively large or if the calf on examination is not in the normal position or presentation.

(10) If the calf can be seen at the vulva and two front legs and head are not presented.

(11) If there are signs of foetal faeces or blood or blood-stained fluid in the vagina or expelled through the vulva.

(12) If the first water bag (allantochorion) lining appears to have separated from the uterus.

If there is any doubt in stockperson's mind as to what is happening or there are any signs of damage to the cow or the calf appears to be too large or the positioning is wrong and outside the competence of the person to rectify, ***then the veterinary surgeon should be called at once***. More cows and calves are lost because of delaying the call for assistance than from calling the veterinarian out too early. It should be remembered that at the start of lactation the cow is at her most valuable. Problems at calving could damage her for the rest of that lactation or cause her premature exit from the herd.

4.4 Abortion

There is considerable variation in the duration of pregnancy (gestation length) in the cow. Gestation usually lasts about 283 days. It is often longer when the calf is sired by a large breed such as a continental cross-bred (e.g. Charolais x Holstein) and often it can then be delayed to 290 days or even longer. It is not unusual for heifers to calve earlier than cows and often this also happens when there are twins. A very early calving is considered by law to be an abortion. Thus in all calvings in the United Kingdom which are 270 days or less in duration must be reported to the Divisional Veterinary Manager of Ministry of Agriculture, Fisheries and Food. At present in some circumstances the animal will not be examined unless in later gestation or a dry cow but, if considered a risk, samples will be taken from the cow and calf to determine whether or not the abortion was due to *Brucella abortus*. It is always a wise move to have each abortion checked for its cause especially if the herd is not closed or there is direct or indirect communication to the cattle on other farms.

There are a large number of different organisms, physical and other causes of abortions for which to be looked. If not done routinely, then if more than two per cent of abortions occur, or two or more cases are close together then they should be checked.

4.5 Examination of the calving cow

On farm, vaginal or uterine examination should only be undertaken if the stockperson is competent, there is sufficient help and an adequate method to restrain the cow. As the cow at calving can be unpredictable, **there should always be two people present** when an examination is to be performed or at least someone should be informed of what is being done and within distance to be called if necessary. This second option is not satisfactory and the former is preferred. The cow is best restrained for such examination between a wall and a gate hinged to the adjacent right angle wall and about 60 cm (two feet) from the corner. If this is not possible, a halter tied to a ring, gate, pole or other fitting which is solid should be adequate. The act of haltering may however distress a cow which is not used to such a procedure and lead to a risk of injury to the cow or the stockperson. Any halter should be attached to the fixed point with a quick release knot. It is not always possible to predict all the likely problems which may be encountered and whether the cow will be distressed by the intervention and so it is always best to have at least two people present. Ensure that there is plenty of warm water available and soap. Lubricating fluid or gel and antiseptics should also be available.

All examination should be performed as cleanly as possible and antiseptic should be added to the water. The arm and the vagina, if dry, should have much soap and water and lubrication applied to it. Ideally the examination should be carried out with a rectal glove especially when initially ensuring there is no obvious infection present within the vagina and uterus or the animal is not aborting. However most people perform the calving without such a protection as it is difficult to grasp the parts of the calf and some tactile sensation is lost. The fingers should be cupped and kept together when entering the vagina and while doing the examination and they must always point towards the calf and away from the vaginal and uterine wall so that no damage is done to the cow. All fingernails should be short and thoroughly cleaned before the hands are introduced through the vulva. Any rings or other jewellery should be removed especially if there are any protrusions which might damage the vaginal wall.

When performing the vaginal examination check that the cervix is fully open and the vagina and uterus appear normal. If there are any signs of abnormality or damage then veterinary help should be sought immediately. Next check the calf and the way it is being presented. If all is well the two front legs and the head should be presented together in the pelvis with the feet of the calf just in front of the head. If possible, whether or not the calf is alive, this should be assessed. It is usually easy to know the calf is alive if it moves or kicks. However it is not always possible to tell if it is dead or not as some live calves remain motionless even when given considerable stimulation.

It is also important when examining to ensure that the head and feet belong to the same calf. This can be difficult to determine. However it is usually possible by passing the hand up one leg and ensuring that it is continuous with the shoulder, neck and head and then do the same on the other side. In addition the size of the calf should be assessed to see if it appears to be too large either by checking the circumference of the lower legs or the apparent size of the head. If it does appear to be too big, for the pelvis of the cow, veterinary assistance should be sought. If the calf appears too small and is at the normal gestation length, it could be that there are twins present or the cow had been served again and not recorded or the calf has had some problem during its development which retarded or stunted its growth. If the calf is in the normal position and the cow shows some healthy straining as examination is being undertaken, then all is likely to be well and the cow should be left to continue the labour without assistance. However she should be checked again in about half an hour. If progress at the next examination is continuing, she again should be able to be left and again re-examined after another half hour.

If on vaginal examination the calf's head cannot be palpated and on further examination two legs with a tail between them is found then the calf is more than likely in posterior presentation. It is often difficult to tell if the leg is front or back. However it is reasonably easy if the lowest joints are felt. Thus if the tail is uppermost to the feet and the first joint above the foot when bent and opened moves the leg straight and down and the second joint above the foot moves the leg straight and up (i.e. the opposite to the first joint above the foot) then it is a hind limb. However if both the first and second joints above the foot move the limb in the same direction, it is a front foot

4.6 Dystocia

Dystocia is an abnormal or difficult calving and is a relatively common occurrence in the dairy cow and particularly the heifer. About 50% of cases of difficult calving are the result of a disproportionate size between the calf and the cow's pelvis and another 25% are a result of the calf being wrongly presented. The problems of disproportionate size of calf to cow can be controlled by the farmer. These mechanisms of control fall under three broad headings, the management of the cow pre-service, the management of the cow pre-calving and management of the cow at calving.

Pre-service management can be best described as the procedures used to select the sire. If sires are not matched adequately to the dam then the incidence of disproportionate size calves is increased. The stockman must pay attention to cow size, conformation and breed. Sires for heifers should be selected on the basis of being breed average or less for the score of calving difficulty and any information on calving of heifers should be scrutinised carefully. If the bull is to be of a dairy breed, then only those with a known record of low incidence of dystocia should be used. It has been suggested that some easy calving sires or dairy breeds are not used on heifers because the resultant progeny may itself have dystocia problems in later life. Heifers that are too small (i.e. less than 360 kg or less than 24 months at projected calving date) should not be served. The size and shape of the pelvis has a major effect on the ease of calving. A useful guide is the hook to pin length. Heifers with short hook to pin distances tend to have a higher incidence of dystocia. Management pre-calving is concerned with target condition scores during the dry period, supplementation of magnesium and frequency of observations made immediately prior to calving. Rapid intervention is not recommended unless any of the criteria mentioned under Section 4.3, points 1 to 12 are fulfilled. However close observation during calving can reduce the incidence of death. Management at calving is essential and is the focus of this Chapter.

The other causes are less common and include a failure of the cervix or vagina to properly relax and dilate (about 10%) and the uterus failing to expel the calf due to inertia (about 5%). This last case can be due to many causes especially low circulating calcium levels or, less likely, iodine deficiency. Other causes of dystocia are other maternal abnormalities)including uterine torsion) which again can amount to about 10% and other foetal problems (5%). Dystocia is also associated with retained placenta and endometritis. Dystocia may also lead to a longer period of time from calving to first service and conception interval and therefore an increased number of inseminations. The mechanisms that are associated with such observations are not fully understood but could be related to delayed uterine involution or suppression of secretion of gonadotrophins.

It is not intended to deal with the problems of calving other than in the broadest outline. Thus if an attempt is to be made to deliver the calf it is important to ensure the cow is sufficiently restrained and there is an adequate amount of labour available. There is also a need for a generous supply of warm or hot water and soap and lubrication. As said earlier, there is also a need to add a suitable antiseptic to the water. Any pulling of the calf should not require more than two people exerting a moderate amount of force. It is always best to apply a calving rope to each leg above the fetlock using a running noose and also to apply a rope to the head again with a noose and going around the ears and into the mouth. Each rope should be attached to a piece of a broom handle or other suitable material and the ropes should be kept short. By having each rope on a different handle each of the legs and head can be manipulated independently thereby helping the calf to be eased through the pelvis and the vulva. Traction should be in unison with the abdominal strainings of the cow. It may be necessary to ease the head out of the vulva by gradually easing and stretching it back over the calf's head.

All traction of calves in the correct position should be in a backward and somewhat downward direction to help ease the calf out of the pelvis. If the calf does not come easily through the pelvic canal, it is best to seek professional help before any damage is done. If the calf is posterior presentation, that is, coming backwards, it is important to try and ease it through the pelvis and once the legs are exposed to calve the cow relatively quickly as the blood supply from the placenta to the calf will often be cut off as it becomes pinched off between the chest of the calf and the bony pelvis. Too much force can lead to damage of the cow including bruised or torn vaginal or uterine tissues, haemorrhage from the uterine artery, dislocation of the spine from the pelvis and fractures of the pelvis. Over-exertion can also result in fore or hind limb fractures of the calf which can often be difficult to heal because of circulatory cessation to the skin or underlying vessels supplying the bone. Front leg muscle atrophy can follow radial paralysis and femoral damage can lead to shrinking of the upper limb muscles in the hind legs. Calving aids are often used as a way of reducing labour. However they must always be used extremely carefully. If too much pressure is applied it can damage the cow very easily. Some calving aids have a device to stop excessive pressure being applied but even these can result in problems if inexpertly used.

4.7 Retained placenta

As this condition occurs after calving it will only be mentioned briefly. There are various definitions of this problem. Thus as seen above, the normal expulsion of the placenta forms the third stage of labour. This has usually happened within 12 hours of the calf being born. However, while a definition of a retained placenta has been one which has present for 24 hours or more after the birth, some now consider retention longer than six hours particularly in older cows to be abnormal. While the placenta remains, milk cannot be sold for human consumption and so this results in economic loss, as does the reduction in appetite, which in turn can lead to less milk production. Following the retention, there is often metritis (uterine inflammation) and this can later lead to reduced fertility.

The reason for the problem of retained placenta is not completely known partly because the mechanisms of normal loss are also not well understood. However factors such as abortion, twins, short or long gestation length and induced calvings can affect it, as does dystocia, milk fever, fatty liver, iodine deficiency, vitamin A and E deficiencies, selenium deficiency and general nutrition. Other factors include the season, heredity, breed, the year, the herd, management change and stress.

Treatment is also open to considerable debate and has not changed radically in the last forty years. Most veterinary surgeons now tend to leave the placenta *in situ* unless the animal is obviously ill or there are other reasons for its rapid removal. If it is to be removed manually, and many consider it should not, then it will usually be left for four or more days. Removal is not usually attempted unless the veterinary surgeon can easily peel the placenta away from the raised cotyledons of the uterus. In some instances the cow will be treated with pessaries or injections of antibiotics. Oestrogen hormones have also been used to increase the uterine tone and blood supply. However their use is not allowed under some milk contracts. In other cases oxytocin or prostaglandin have been used and some have tried other ecbolics such as ergot derivatives to eject the recalcitrant placenta. Prevention usually involves the use of oxytocin, prostaglandins or other hormones to hasten their removal, but the actual value of such treatments is not proved. Treatment with antibiotics or oestrogens are often used to reduce the chances of endometritis (inflammation of the uterine lining), but again their benefits are arguable. Gonadotrophin releasing hormone (GnRH) injection after retained placenta has been claimed to reduce endometritis.

4.8 Post-calving coliform mastitis

One of the most common mastitic problems in the recently calved cow is environmental mastitis particularly caused by *Escherichia coli*. Table 4.1 shows the proportions of the various pathogens present in the samples from cows with mastitis. It can be seen that *E. coli* forms the largest percentage of isolates in recent years.

Table 4.1 The number and percentage distribution of pathogens in milk samples examined by the Veterinary Investigation Service, UK from 1992 to 1998 (VIDA, 1999).

Organism	1992	1993	1994	1995	1996	1997	1998	Av. 93-98
E. coli	29.1	27.5	28.7	28.5	28.1	26.4	26.3	27.6
S. uberis	17.8	18.4	17.6	17.3	18.7	21.6	22.4	19.3
Coagulase + ve staphs.	17.5	16.3	15.9	19.1	18.6	19.6	18.8	18.1
S. dysgalactiae	9.7	8.6	8.1	7.3	7.3	6.1	5.7	7.2
A. pyogenes	5.0	4.8	4.8	3.4	3.3	2.8	2.6	3.6
S. agalactiae	4.8	5.1	5.2	4.7	3.4	2.1	1.5	3.7
Other pathogens	16.1	13	12.8	12.6	11.5	12.3	12.3	12.3
No pathogens	NR	6.1	7.1	7.2	9.1	9.7	10.3	8.2
No. of isolates	5404	6006	6592	7311	6089	6894	6050	-

Many of these infections occur in the first month after calving, and most veterinary surgeons and farmers consider that all coliform infections are very severe with a very sick animal and marked udder swelling. However although *E. coli* infections do cause the largest proportion of severe infections in cows, this type of mastitis is not the most common expression of the disease even with this bacterium (see Table 4.2)

Table 4.2 The relative distribution of pathogens and their clinical severity

Pathogen	Very Severe	Severe	Mild
E. coli	14.3%	35.3%	50.5%
S.uberis	6.0%	35.6%	58.4%
Staphylococci	3.4%	23.8%	72.8%
S.dysgalactiae	7.2%	38.4%	54.4%
S.agalactiae	6.7%	34.1%	59.2%
All cases	7.6%	29.8%	62.6%

Source: Veterinary Record (1980)

It is very unusual to see coliform mastitis in the dry period and when it does occur most cases will be very close to calving. Studies have shown that 20.8% of *E. coli* mastitis cases are seen at calving and another 22.9% occur in the next five weeks. The reason for the very low level in the dry cow and rapid rise after calving depends on the nature of the coliform infection and the cow's own defense mechanisms. Usually *E. coli* organisms do not remain in the udder as a persistent source of infection. Thus under normal circumstances, they enter the udder via the teat canal and either are eliminated rapidly by the host's defense mechanisms or cause mastitis within about two days of their entry. Only a very small proportion of cows are carriers of the infection.

The quiescent dry udder has a very high level of natural resistance to *E. coli* and some other infections. This is largely due to a defense mechanism known as the lactoferrin/citrate/bicarbonate system which operates in the dry udder. When actively multiplying *E. coli* organisms require iron to be readily available. However in the dry udder there are large quantities of lactoferrin, which is a large molecule protein that binds with almost all the available iron present within the udder. This effectively prevents the *E. coli* from multiplying and produces an unfavourable environment for the bacterium.

4.9 Diapedesis and toxic shock

Immediately before calving, the environment in the udder changes and there is an increase in citrate ions in the udder secretion. These compete with lactoferrin causing the release of iron which is then made available for bacterial growth. Thus in the few days before calving or immediately afterwards the udder becomes very vulnerable should *E. coli* enter. If coliforms are introduced, then one of two major scenarios can occur.

(1) When the defence mechanisms are working satisfactorily white cells called phagocytes enter the udder and engulf and destroy the invading organisms. This process of entry is called diapedesis and when it is working satisfactorily the number of white cells in the milk and milk forming tissues will increase rapidly by 40 to 250 fold.

(2) However often in the freshly calved cow diapedesis is slow or delayed and so bacteria can rapidly multiply in a favourable environment resulting in potent toxin production and disease. These toxins result in increasing the permeability of the blood vessels leading to fluid accumulation in the udder (oedema), rapid acute swelling of one or more quarters. This is then followed by a delayed but rapid rise in the number of cells in the milk.

If diapedesis is delayed there can be very rapid multiplication and build-up of bacteria in the udder and toxin production. This can result in the milk showing no visible changes but the effects of the toxins and the inflammatory processes occurring will result in a very sick animal. They all contribute to a rapidly developing syndrome. Thus the cow can initially show a complete loss of appetite, temperature rise and muscle trembling. Some animals also develop a severe watery diarrhoea. As the toxins rise still further a typical toxic shock syndrome develops with a fall in temperature to below normal, shivering, pale and cold nose and mouth, weakness and then rapid collapse. It is often then not long before the animal becomes comatosed and dies.

The consequences of this condition are variable and a large number of cows will die despite adequate treatment. Probably deaths are now slightly fewer than a few years ago due to improved therapy and farmers realising the severity of the condition and so undertaking therapy promptly. However, of those that survive, little work has been undertaken to follow them up during the lactation. Work in the United States of America showed that of cows with severe coliform mastitis which survived, 60% of cows returned to produce milk, in the affected quarter that lactation, and of these 11% were subsequently culled in that lactation, half because of low milk yield. In the 40% which failed to return to milk in that quarter that lactation, 11% remained in the herd and half of these had milk in the affected quarter the next lactation.

4.10 Treatment of coliform mastitis

For treatment to be effective in coliform or toxic mastitis, it needs to be undertaken early and thoroughly. It will require the assistance of the veterinary surgeon. There are still many different opinions on how to treat, but all are agreed on the need to treat the shock and the various breakdown products from the bacteria and white cells. This is done usually by the veterinary surgeon giving an anti-inflammatory agent such as the non-steroidal anti-inflammatory agents flunixin, ketoprofen, meloxicam or carprofen. Some veterinary surgeons may give a large dose of corticosteroids to again assist with the shock. Many will also give fluids intravenously to counteract the tissue dehydration which occurs, this may be in the form of isotonic saline or other fluids which are in the same concentration as in the blood. Recently, the use of hypertonic saline has found favour. This highly concentrated solution of salt which is usually given in about a three litre volume over a short period of time. The aim is that as the injection is concentrated, it will draw fluid back into the blood. In addition the cow will show thirst and should be offered and have easy access to water. Many cows which are recumbent will often get to their feet within a few minutes of the injection.

The long term results of such therapy have not been fully evaluated as yet but when a cow is treated by a veterinary surgeon, a second visit should be undertaken to assess progress within 24 hours or much less. Antibiotic injections are usually given with the aim of killing off the bacteria but their effects may be variable. Intramammary antibiotics are also used but in many instances they are of limited help as the main problem is the toxin which is produced. Much more important is to bathe and massage the udder and try to remove as much of the fluid present within as possible as this contains the toxins which will otherwise be absorbed into the animal and result in her becoming even more ill. The more often the quarters are drawn the more likely the animal is to recover.

4.11 Prevention of coliform mastitis

Preventive advice is easier said than done. All cattle should be kept in a clean environment. This is particularly important during the last part of pregnancy and the first month of lactation. This means all calving boxes must be kept clean and generously supplied with clean dry straw or other appropriate bedding material. It should be ensured that there are sufficient calving boxes for the number of cows likely to calve at a time. The cow should ideally remain in this clean environment for the first few days after calving. Cubicles, if used following calving, should be of the correct measurements for the particular cow. Length, width, head and side rail should all be of the correct size for the cow.

The bedding used should be comfortable, warm and in sufficient quantity. In most instances it should be chopped straw and if not sand is useful although not as warm as straw or soft wood shavings which contain natural oils to reduce bacterial multiplication. Shredded paper or rubber mats can also be useful. Mattresses filled with shredded tyres or water could be suitable but they need more evaluation. All damp or soiled bedding should be removed at least twice daily. If straw yards are used then they again should be kept clean and dry. This means that bedding should be used generously. All lying areas must be of sufficient size and be comfortable and draught-free. Ideally, all freshly calved cows should spend a time in a straw yard until they are settled to their diet and routine.

The production of loose faeces can increase its coliform count and this can often happen with the change of feeding which occurs at calving. It is therefore desirable to include straw in the feed to improve the digestion of the material and ensure a more firm form of faeces with a reduced coliform count. Pre-milking hygiene is important and clipping the hair on the tail and udder will keep the latter cleaner.

All cows which milk out quickly tend to have more open teat sphincters after milking and so all cows should not be allowed to go back to their cubicles or straw yard immediately after milking. If they lie down and the sphincter is still relaxed it will make it that much more easy for pathogens to enter the teat canal. Thus it is sound advice to allow the cows to stand for a period of about half an hour after milking to allow teat sphincter closure. This is often best achieved by providing a loafing area for the cows before their return to the cubicles with provision of food in this area.

Pre-milking hygiene is important and the animals should be kept as clean as possible between milkings. If the teats are dirty then they should be cleaned and then dried to ensure that no contaminated material congregates at the teat end. In some herds where environmental mastitis has been a problem, pre-milking teat dipping has proved useful. This involves cleaning, if necessary, the teats and then applying a disinfectant before its removal and then milking the cow. This does not stop the need for post milking teat dipping. Teat dipping after milking is an important part of the prevention of contagious mastitis organisms. However it is of very limited help in the prevention of environmental mastitis, although the prolonged use of certain dips will produce a gradual decrease in the level of environmental mastitis in the herd.

An *E. coli* J5 vaccine has been available in North America for many years. It is now being introduced to the UK for control of this problem. While it does not prevent all cases of *E. coli* infection, it will reduce the number and severity of problems in most herds annually where the disease is prevalent. The preventive programme involves a course of three injections and vaccination must be used as an addition and not to replace normal *E. coli* preventative measures.

4.12 Peracute staphylococcal mastitis

This, like the peracute toxic coliform mastitis, occurs soon after calving. It is by far the least common of the staphylococcal forms (Table 4.2), but is the one requiring the most concentrated effort to control. For every case of peracute staphylococcal mastitis there are probably six or seven peracute *E. coli* cases. The reason for staphylococci causing this type of mastitis is unknown. It is possible to create mastitis experimentally by injecting *Staphylococcus aureus* into the udder. However there is a great variation in the severity of disease and this is not just the result of the virulence of the organisms used. The problem does appear to worsen in cattle in early lactation. Following disease there are circulating antibodies to *S. aureus* although these do not appear to protect the cow from further attack. However the peracute form can be produced experimentally in the udder of a cow later in lactation by removing all the antibody present within the mammary gland. Much of the available circulating antibody enters the udder during the late dry period to be concentrated in the colostrum and then is lost to the cow. It is thus possible that the circulating antibody does have some effect in controlling infection and its reduction allows the more severe toxic and dangerous form of reaction to occur.

The peracute form of staphylococcal mastitis usually occurs in the first few days after calving. The cow is severely affected with signs of sudden onset. There is profound depression, a very high temperature, usually 41° to 42°C (106° to 108°F), complete loss of appetite, static gut and muscle weakness often resulting in recumbency. An animal can be completely normal at one milking and nearly dead by the next. The mammary gland will have one or more quarters swollen, hot, hard and painful. The fluid drawn from the affected teat is often watery and reddish-brown in colour. Other unaffected quarters will usually be swollen with oedema (fluid under the skin). In some there is also fluid accumulation in front of the udder. There is often lameness on the side of swelling and, in some cases, the stifle and hock can be swollen. Often, in a few hours, the quarter develops a red to purple/black colour usually starting at the base of the teat and spreading over the floor of the udder. In some animals blisters form. The area becomes cold and clammy to the touch and often will start to ooze clear yellow serum. At this stage little or no fluid can be drawn from the udder and if fluid can be drawn it is blood-stained and watery without clots or smell.

The cow becomes more and more ill (toxic) and in many cases she will die. If she does survive, she will loose the quarter and often the skin will separate from the underlying tissues and be shed with often part of the udder tissue. In other cases the inner part of the udder will separate later and will detach unless helped to do so in a period of weeks or months. The shed material and that remaining is often covered by a thin layer of pus and the remains of the quarter will heal over a period of several more weeks.

The acute form of *Staphylococcus aureus* infection is also more commonly seen in early lactation and is not as dramatic as the peracute form. There may in such cases be some rise in temperature but only up to 39.5° to 40°C (103° to 104°F) at the most. The quarter is swollen, and reddened and drawing the teat produces milk which is purulent or contains thick clots. Following recovery there is extensive thickening within the udder tissue resulting in reduced or loss of milk production.

Treatment of the peracute staphylococcal infections in many ways is very similar to that for peracute *E. coli* infections and involves counteracting the toxic shock often using anti-inflammatory agents. Your veterinary surgeon will need to be called. Non steroidal anti-inflammatory agents are used or one, or a few, large doses of corticosteroids. Fluid therapy is also often essential and again isotonic or hypertonic saline can be used. Antibiotics can be injected and, for the most part, different ones will be required to those for coliform infections. Intramammary tube use may be of some help but often the swelling will prevent good distribution of the antibiotic. If there is no gangrene present, the quarter should be stripped as often as practicable to remove as much of the toxin as possible.

Prevention is to undertake suitable dry cow therapy and to try and ensure the nutrition and management of the animal is conducive to preventing stress and trying to maintain at a high level the animal's ability to respond to disease.

4.13 Other causes of post-calving mastitis

Several other bacteria can cause mastitis in the immediate period post calving. As can be seen from Table 4.1, *Streptococcus uberis* infection is becoming more common and often mimics *E. coli* problems. It is essential to find out the cause of these severe cases so that appropriate management strategies can be initiated. Generalising, *S. uberis* infection is most commonly seen when straw is used as bedding. It is essential where this bacterium is the major cause of the mastitis that all straw bedding is kept absolutely dry and generously supplied. Therapy is normally reasonably similar to that for *E. coli* mastitis. Other environmental pathogens occasionally seen include *Klebsiella, Pseudomonas and Bacillis cereus* as well as many other organisms. Most of these again, tend to be similar to *E. coli.* Occasionally streptococcal infections will cause severe disease at this time and treatment and control tend to be similar to that for *S. aureus.*

Further recommended reading

Albright, J.L. and Arawe, C.W. (1997) *The Behaviour of Cattle.* CAB International, Wallingford, UK.

Andrews, A.H. (1990) *Outline of Clinical Diagnosis in Cattle.* Wright, London, UK.

Andrews, A.H. (2000) *The Health of Dairy Cattle.* Blackwell Sciences Ltd, Oxford, UK.

Edwards, W.A. (1980) Mastitis Surveillance Scheme January to June 1980. *Veterinary Record* **107**, 297.

Noakes, D.J. (1986) *Fertility and Obstetrics in Cattle.* Blackwell Sciences Ltd., Oxford, UK.

VIDA (1999) *Veterinary Investigation Surveillance Report* 1998 and 1991 to 1998. Veterinary Laboratory Agency, Weybridge, UK.

Chapter 5
FEEDING STRATEGIES

5.1 Introduction

The dry period is not a period of rest for the expectant cow. It is a period of dynamic change - a period of preparation for the rigours of the next lactation. Nutrition of the expectant cow is therefore an important subject and the development of nutritional management plans will prevent mistakes that can affect the welfare of the cow and be costly in financial terms. It is difficult to rectify mistakes in nutrition during late pregnancy by any modifications to the diet as the dry period is of limited duration. Therefore the nutrition of the cow during late lactation is important and is considered integral to the feeding strategy of the expectant cow. Inappropriate nutrition of the cow during the dry period can compromise the establishment of high yields of milk in lactation and may impair fertility. Why therefore has the nutritional management of the expectant cow been neglected, or has it been neglected? This chapter attempts to map the major advances in the nutritional management and provides a "blue-print" which we hope many of the readers feel to be the correct formula for the cow.

The authors have used the same notation and same equations as outlined in *"Energy and Protein Requirements of Ruminants"* by the Technical Committee on Responses to Nutrients, published by CAB International for the Agricultural and Food Research Council (AFRC, 1993).

5.2 Theoretical considerations

To understand the changes in the nutrition of the cow in late pregnancy, it is necessary to understand some of the basic considerations that have to be accounted when constructing diets. Weighing of cattle is an essential pre-requisite to diet formulation. Two methods are available on-farm, the calibrated weigh crush (which is quite rare) and the weigh-band. The weigh-band is a simple tool which can provide a relatively accurate assessment of the animal's live-weight (probably within 20 to 30 kg of actual weight). The majority of the discussion in this Chapter will concentrate on rationing a cow carrying one calf. Cows carrying multiple foetuses have an increase in their requirement for energy, protein and minerals, but they have a lower capacity to eat feed. This poses significant problems and adds yet another complexity to the process of rationing. The dry period should be subdivided into two parts - the "far-off or early dry period" (56 to 21 days before calving) and the "close-up or late dry period" (21 days to calving).

5.3 Voluntary feed intake of cows during late pregnancy

The voluntary feed intake of the cow is probably the most important management tool available to the nutritionist. The limits to voluntary feed intake have been classified as animal factors (rumen capacity, milk yield and fatness) and feed factors (chemical composition, water content) and the interaction between the factors. The voluntary intake of cows during the dry period usually ranges between 12 and 14 kg dry matter (DM) per day (1.8 to 2.0% of live weight). It is important to maintain the voluntary intake of cows throughout the whole dry period, but during the last 5 to 7 days, the voluntary intake of the cow declines rapidly. The main reason for the decline in intake is complex but could be related to the size of the developing calf and the pregnant uterus, changes in physiological control of intake and behavioural reasons. Intake of feed during the last 5 to 7 days of pregnancy may be as low as 7 to 9 kg DM per day (about 30% reduction in intake; about 1.3% of live weight) and therefore the ration (especially the energy density) may need altering. If changes in formulation are to be incorporated into the system of feeding, sources of forage and concentrate must be highly palatable as well as having greater concentrations of energy and possibly protein.

Table 5.1 Effect of digestibility of forage and level of concentrate offered on total DM intakes (kg/day) of cows in late pregnancy.

Live weight (kg)	Concentrate (kg DM/day)	Forage D-value (g/kg DM) 550	600	650	700	750
550	0	6.9	8.7	10.4	12.2	14.0
	2	7.8	9.6	11.6	13.1	14.9
600	0	7.4	9.3	11.1	13.0	na
	2	8.2	10.1	12.0	13.9	na
650	0	7.8	9.8	11.8	13.8	na
	2	8.6	10.6	12.6	14.6	na
700	0	8.3	10.4	12.5	14.6	na
	2	9.0	11.1	13.2	15.3	na

na - not applicable

There are no official recommendations in the United Kingdom for the voluntary intake of cows during late pregnancy. The digestibility of the forage offered (the main component of the ration) to any classification of ruminant affects the voluntary intake of the feed. Also, the intake and the appetite of the cow is affected by the level of concentrate offered with the forage (Table 5.1). The equation used to calculate the forage DM intake of dry cows is:

Forage DMI (kg/day) = (0.0003111[DOMD] - 0.00478C - 0.1102)W0.75
where

DOMD is the digestibility of digestible organic matter (D-value) reported as g/kg and not%.
C is the DM intake of concentrate
W is the live weight of the cow

After the forage DM intake has been calculated, the intake of concentrate DM must be added to calculate the total DM intake.

The voluntary intakes of feed for various classifications of dairy cow during late pregnancy recommended by researchers in the United States are:

	Stage of dry period	
	"Far-off period"	"Close-up period"
	Feed intake (g DM/kg W)	
Heifers	18.5	15.0
Mature cows	21.0	17.5
Twin pregnancies	19.0	15.0

Source: NRC (1989)

Accessibility to feed rather than the actual level of nutrients available in the feed may be more important during the period to 21 days prior to calving. Competition for feed and water is an important consideration when housing and managing dry cows in groups. In general the same rules apply as for lactating cows; that is about 75 cm per cow at the feed trough and a cow density of no more than 1 cow per 7 m^2. If these rules are broken for any reason, a restriction in voluntary intake and hence nutrient intake may occur.

The development of a social hierachy within loose yards of dry cows can also be observed with dominant multiparous cows feeding before heifers. As a result, cows and heifers with a lower social dominance will either receive a ration which may be restricted in quantity or they will have to increase their rate of eating. Multiparous cows also consume more dry matter per meal over a shorter period of time than heifers. They also ruminate more with a greater efficiency and drink more water. Therefore in order to ensure heifers and cows of lower social dominance receive adequate levels of feed, greater levels of feed must be offered with a reduction in competitive pressure at the feed trough. This could work against any plans of restricting voluntary intake if cows have mixed or excessive condition.

In a detailed study of social and feeding behaviour of cows during the last two weeks of pregnancy, it was found that about 48% of time was spent resting, 16% eating, 25% ruminating and 11% of time spent showing other behaviour for example drinking, grooming and vocalising. In contrast lactating cows spend 21% of each day eating, 32% of time ruminating, 33% of time was spent resting and 14% of time in other behavioural activities. Both series of data suggest the rate of eating by the cows was not restricted and therefore the cow would easily ensure her intake of feed met her target for production.

5.4 Energy requirement

The energy requirement of the cow in the dry period is the sum of her requirements for maintenance, pregnancy and growth (if the cow is in her first or second lactation). The method of rationing is known as the factorial model. This calculation of energy requirement is nearly equal to the cows' requirement for maintenance plus 4 to 8 litres of milk per day.

The formula to calculate the metabolisable energy requirement (MER) of a cow in late pregnancy is:

$$\text{MER (MJ/day)} = \text{Mm} + \text{Mc}$$

Eqn. 1

where Mm = maintenance requirement (MJ/day)
Mc = pregnancy requirement (MJ/day)

If however the animal being considered is a heifer or possibly in her second lactation, she will also have a requirement for energy to grow. Therefore:

MER (MJ/day) = Mm + Mc + Mg Eqn. 2

where Mc and Mm are as in Equation 1 and
Mg = requirement for growth (MJ/day)

The calculation of requirements of metabolisable energy for maintenance (Mm) is broken down into two components, fasting metabolism (F) and activity allowance (A).

Therefore: $F\ (MJ/day) = 0.53\ (W/1.08)^{0.67}$ Eqn.3
A (MJ/day) = 0.0095W Eqn.4

and Mm (MJ/day) = (F + A)/km Eqn.5

where W = live weight of the cow
km = efficiency of utilisation of metabolisable energy for maintenance (km = 0.72).

The calculations made below have allowed for a safety margin and 5% has been added for the purpose of rationing. **It is essential that all rations for all classifications of cattle should be examined by a suitably qualified nutritionist and that all feedingstuffs are analysed before being used in a ration.**

Example 1. A 600 kg cow (second lactation) has a fasting requirement (F) of 36.6 MJ/day (Equation 3) and an activity allowance (A; Equation 4) of 5.7 MJ/day. The calculation of total maintenance requirement for this cow is set out in Equation 5 and is 58.8 MJ/day. This total for maintenance should be increased by 5% to take into account a safety margin for the purpose of rationing. The maintenance requirement (MER) of this cow is therefore 61.7 MJ/day or 62 MJ/day.

The requirement for pregnancy assumes the total energy retained in the gravid uterus at a designated time (t) during pregnancy is:

$$\log_{10}(E_t) = 151.665 - 151.64e^{-0.0000576t} \qquad \text{Eqn.6}$$

where t is days from conception (assuming the calf weighs 40 kg at birth)

The energy retained daily (Ec) can be calculated by

$$E_c\ (\text{MJ/day}) = 0.025W_c\ (E_t \times 0.0201e^{-0.0000576t}) \qquad \text{Eqn.7}$$

where Et in MJ is the energy retained in the gravid uterus
W_m is the birth weight of the calf (kg)

The birth-weight of the calf can be calculated from the following formula

$$W_c = (W_m{}^{0.73} - 28.89) / 2.064 \qquad \text{Eqn.8}$$

where W_m is the mature body weight of the cow

Example 2. The cow mentioned in Example 1, weighing 600kg and had a calculated total maintenance requirement of 61.7 MJ/day. The estimated weight of the calf at full-term from this cow would be 37.7 kg (Equation 8).

These calculations lead to the following energy requirements for cows at different stages of pregnancy (Table 5.2) and at differing live weights (Table 5.3).

Table 5.2 Requirement for metabolisable energy to support pregnancy (assuming a 40 kg calf)

	Weeks Pregnant								
	25	30	32	34	36	37	38	39	40
MJ/day	5.5	11.1	14.6	19.2	25.4	29.1	33.5	38.4	44.1

Source: AFRC (1993)

Table 5.3 Requirement for metabolisable energy to support maintenance (MJ/day).

Live-weight (kg)	400	450	500	550	600	650	700	750
Mm (MJ/day)	46	50	55	58	62	65	69	69

Source: AFRC (1993)

Table 5.4 Calf birth-weight (kg) by breed (pure breed)

Angus	26	Guernsey	33
Ayrshire	35	Holstein	45
Friesian	39	Jersey	26

Source: AFRC (1993)

It has been assumed that the energy requirement for pregnancy is directly related to the birth-weight of the calf. Therefore to correct the energy requirement for pregnancy the ratio of expected birth-weight to 40kg should be implemented. However not all pure breed calves are 40 kg and a correction factor must be calculated (Table 5.4). For example if a Holstein calf weighing 45 kg is born, the requirement of energy to support pregnancy should be corrected by a factor of 45/40 or 1.125.

The calculations of energy requirement for growth in the heifer during late pregnancy are difficult to make. It is correct to use the equation for energy requirement of the growing heifer, treating the heifer as an animal which may be used for beef production or herd replacement (that is when the animal is still less than 400 kg) or do we consider the calculations which consider live-weight change in lactating cattle? Lean tissue deposition requires about 5 MJ/kg DM of actual muscle but the deposition of fat requires about 39 MJ/kg DM.

The energy value ascribed to weight gains of heifers for medium size breeds (for example Friesian or Holstein-Friesian) is as follows:

$$\text{Energy value of gain} = \frac{1.30\,(4.1 + 0.0332W - 0.000009W^2)}{(1 - 0.1475\,\Delta W)} \qquad \text{Eqn. 9}$$

where W = live-weight of the heifer

ΔW = the change in live-weight of the heifer

Example 3. By using this equation the energy requirement for a 450 kg heifer with a live-weight change of 0.5 kg/day would be 24.2 MJ/day. If the live weight change of the cow is used to estimate the requirement for growth then the allowance of net energy for empty-body weight live-weight change in mature dairy cattle is 19 MJ/kg increase and a release of 16 MJ/kg to metabolism for 1 kg loss.

In the United States, the requirement for growth in the pregnant heifer is considered by adding another 20% of the total energy requirement to the ration of the dry heifer. This may be a compromise but would at term for a 500 kg heifer equate to approximately 19 MJ/day for growth.

5.4.1 How to formulate a ration for energy

Rationing the cow for her requirement for metabolisable energy is relatively simple and best explained using an example.

Example 4. What are the requirements for metabolisable energy for a 600 kg cow in the last week of pregnancy (week 40) neither gaining or losing live-weight and assuming the birth-weight of the calf is 40 kg?

M_m (Table 5.2)	59 MJ/day
Pregnancy (Table 5.2)	44 MJ/day
sub total	103 MJ/day
Add 5% safety margin	5 MJ/day
Total requirement	**108 MJ/day**

The key to accurate rationing of a cow is to ensure the level of metabolisable energy eaten is equal to the requirement. If the cow above is fed 35 kg of grass silage (22% dry matter and 10.6 MJ/kg DM), how much concentrate containing 11.0 MJ/kg DM (85% DM) is required to ensure the cow is fed to requirement?

	As fed offered	DM content	ME offered	ME
Grass silage	35 kg	7.7 kg	10.6 MJ/kgDM	81.6 MJ
Concentrate	XX kg	X.X kg	11.0MJ/kgDM	XX.X MJ
Total requirement				**108 MJ**

To solve the problem, the cow would require a further 26.4 MJ/day (81.6 + 26.4 = 108MJ) to ensure the requirements for maintenance and pregnancy are fulfilled. Therefore:

26.4/11.0 = kg of concentrate DM/day required
= 2.4 kg DM/day

Assuming the DM of the concentrate is 85%, then

2.4/ (85/100) = 2.8 kg of concentrate as fed

Can the cow eat this level of feed? The total DM intake was calculated as 7.7 + 2.4 = 10.1 kg DM/day. A cow in the last week of pregnancy can eat about 1.8% of her body-weight or 10.8 kg DM/day. The diet is therefore sufficient in energy and also can be eaten by the cow.

5.5 Protein requirement

The system used currently to calculate the requirements and therefore to ration the animal is known as the Metabolisable Protein System or MP system. The system is outlined in detail in AFRC (1993). The general philosophy to calculate the requirements is similar to that used to calculate requirements for metabolisable energy but when calculating the ration, the system considers the level of energy available to the microbial population in the rumen (fermentable metabolisable energy, FME) as well as how fast the protein breaks down in the rumen (the degradability of the protein; the so-called level of eRDP (effective rumen degradable protein) and DUP, digestible but undegradable protein - not available to rumen bacteria.

The maintenance requirements for metabolisable protein (MPm) are calculated by the sum of the net protein requirements for basal endogenous protein requirement and dermal losses in scurf and hair (Table 5.5).

$$\text{MPm (g/day)} = 2.30W^{0.75} \qquad \text{Eqn. 10}$$

The requirements for pregnancy are based on the daily retention of protein in the tissue of the calf (NPc):

$$NP_c \text{ (g/day)} = TP_t \times 34.37e^{-0.00262t} \qquad \text{Eqn. 11}$$

where t is the number of days from conception and TPt is calculated as:

$$\log_{10}(TP_t) = 3.707 - 5.698e^{-0.00262t} \qquad \text{Eqn. 12}$$

The values for NPc and TPt are based on the projected birth-weight of the calf being 40 kg in a similar fashion to that for the calculation of energy requirement. The metabolisable protein requirement of pregnancy (Table 5.6) is therefore:

$$\text{MP (g/day)} = 1.01W_c(TP_t \times e^{-0.00262t}) \qquad \text{Eqn. 13}$$

The calculations for metabolisable protein requirements for growth suffer from the same complexities as the calculations for energy requirement. In the case of growing pregnant heifers (or possible cows in their second lactation) the metabolisable protein requirement is:

$$MPf\ (g/day) = 0.80\ (168.07 - 0.16869W + 0.0001633W^2) \times (1.12 - 0.1223\Delta W) \times 1.695\Delta W \qquad \text{Eqn. 14}$$

where W is the live weight of the heifer and
ΔW is the change in live weight of the heifer during pregnancy

The metabolisable protein requirement for live-weight gain in mature cows is 233 g MP/day. The level of metabolisable protein released when 1 kg of live-weight of lost by a mature cow is 138 g/day.

Table 5.5 Metabolisable protein requirements for maintenance

Live-weight	**MPm** (g/day)
400	216
450	236
500	256
550	275
600	293
650	312
700	329
750	347

Source: AFRC (1993)

Table 5.6 Requirement for metabolisable protein to support pregnancy (assuming a 40 kg calf)

Weeks pregnant	**Requirement** (g/day)
25	34
30	64
32	82
34	102
36	127
37	141
38	156
39	173
40	191

Source: AFRC(1993)

5.5.1 How to formulate a ration for protein

The first calculation to be made is to determine the animal production level (APL) for the cow. This is calculated as:

$$APL = ME_{\mathbf{total}} / ME_{maintenance} \qquad \text{Eqn. 15}$$

In the case of a cow in the final week of pregnancy, we have calculated her total requirement for metabolisable energy in the previous section.

$$APL = 108/59 = 1.83 \qquad \text{Eqn. 16}$$

A feed composition table is required to determine the relevant concentrations of eRDP that each feed offered in the ration can provide.

If we take, as an example the ration offered to the dry cow in Section 5.3.1 on rationing for metabolisable energy (Example 4), we can gain the following information from feed tables and chemical analysis.

	Crude protein (g/kg DM)	eRDP (g/kg DM)	DUP (g/kg DM)	FME (MJ/kg DM)
Grass silage	140	99.3	13.4	7.6
Concentrate	207	144.8	37.5	9.9

The amount of eRDP in the ration is the level available for rumen bacteria to use, but it is little use to offer the rumen bacteria protein only. A supply of metabolisable energy which can be broken down in the rumen must be present for microbial crude protein to be formed.

The amount of eRDP offered in the ration is the level of eRDP multiplied by the DM intake of each feed.

Grass silage	99.3 x 7.7	=	764.6 g/day
Concentrate	144.8 x 2.8	=	405.4 g/day
Total eRDP (g/day)		=	1170 g/day

This energy source is known as fermentable metabolisable energy (FME) and is generally reported on analytical results sheets for silage and in tables of feed composition for concentrates. The amount of FME provided by the ration is

Grass silage	7.6 x 7.7	=	58.5 MJ/day
Concentrate	9.9 x 2.8	=	27.7 MJ/day
Total FME (MJ/day)		=	86.2 MJ/day

The level of microbial crude protein (MCP) can be limited either by a lack of eRDP or a lack of FME. The next step to ration the cow is to see which source is lacking (if any). If eRDP is lacking the level of MCP that can be formed is exactly equal to the level of eRDP.

$$\text{MCP}_{\text{(protein limited)}} = \text{eRDP} = 1170 \text{ g/day}$$

The level of animal production (APL) affects the amount of microbial yield. Therefore:

$$\text{MCP}_{\text{(energy limited)}} = 9.8 \times 86.2 = 845 \text{ g/day}$$

The smaller of the two values of MCP is the one for energy limited (845 g/day vs. 1170 g/day). Therefore the yield of MCP is limited by FME. When the dry cow is given the ration containing grass silage and concentrate 845 g of microbial crude protein will be leaving the rumen each day.

Only 0.75 of the microbial protein is true protein (available to the ruminant) and the cow is only able to absorb 85% of the true protein synthesised by the bacteria. Therefore the level of microbial true protein (MTP) available to the cow is 64% of that synthesised. Thus:

$$\text{MTP} = 845 \times 0.64 = 541\text{g/day}$$

The cow has another source of protein in the feed available to her to convert to metabolisable protein. We have calculated the level of microbial crude protein available for conversion to metabolisable protein and we must add the level of feed digestible but undegradable protein (DUP).

The level of DUP available from the ration each day is

DUP (g/day) = Grass silage: 7.7 x 13.4 = 103.2
DUP (g/day) = Concentrate: 2.8 x 37.5 = 105.0
= 208.2 g/day

Therefore the MP supplied by DUP or "by-pass" protein is 208 g/day.

The total supply of metabolisable protein to the cow is calculated as:

$$\text{MP}_{(\text{total})} = \text{MTP} + \text{DUP}$$

$$\text{MP}_{(\text{total})} = 541 + 208 = 749 \text{ g/day.}$$

The calculation for the requirement of the cow for metabolisable protein has been outlined in a previous section. The cow in the rationing example was 600 kg and at full-term (40 weeks of gestation). Her requirements for metabolisable protein are:

MPR (g/day) = MPm + MPc

MPR (g/day) = 293 + 191 = 584 g/day (Tables 5.5 and 5.6).

The diet provides 749 g of metabolisable protein per day and the cow requires 584 g/day. Therefore the ration supplies a surplus of 165 g MP/day. The cow would either excrete the surplus or potentially she could de-aminate the protein and use it as a source of metabolisable energy. The latter process may well be an important factor in the feeding of the over-conditioned cow up to the "close-up" dry period. It is also interesting to note that the cow required 43 g of the DUP supplied by the ration, but the surplus metabolisable protein should not be considered as solely DUP and therefore no reduction in the supply of DUP should be made when rationing the cow.

5.6 Mineral nutrition

Fourteen different minerals are required to a greater or lesser degree to maintain good health and productive function of ruminants. These minerals are sub divided into two classes, the major minerals which are required in relatively large amounts such as calcium (Ca), phosphorus (P) and magnesium (Mg) and the trace elements required in very much smaller quantities such as copper (Cu), zinc (Zn), selenium (Se) and iron (Fe).

The diagnosis of mineral deficiencies is not always straight forward as the signs may well be confused with other metabolic, nutritional or health problems or they are just not specific. In certain instances the clinical signs of a deficiency is specific and therefore the method of correction of the problem is well documented. However in most instances the signs of deficiency or imbalance may not be apparent and corrective action is difficult to implement. The key to accurate and rapid diagnosis of a problem is the keeping of good records. This process is invaluable to the stockperson as it may save valuable time and money and alleviate a problem before it becomes a major one. It will also aid the development of management plans for herds as well as provide information to make strategic decisions.

The requirement of a certain mineral by an animal is determined in a similar fashion to that of energy and protein. It is based on a quantitative factorial model which considers:

First level of model	**Second level of model**
Maintenance	Faecal endogenous loss - that lost from the body via the faeces. Minerals are lost from the body through the gut wall as digestive secretions, via saliva or bile.
	Urine loss - urinary excretion is an essential path to remove excessive levels of minerals from the body. However if the diet is inadequate in its mineral composition, excretion via the urine still occurs (albeit at a reduced level) and may result in a further reduction in the overall mineral balance.
Production	Tissue deposition (growth) Pregnancy Milk production

The maintenance and production requirements when added together are the *net requirement* of the animal for the mineral. A calculation of the gross requirement for the mineral is necessary to formulate a ration (dietary allowance) which provides an adequate level for maintenance and production.

$$\text{Gross requirement} = \frac{\text{net requirement}}{\text{absorption coefficient}}$$

$$\text{Dietary allowance} = \frac{\text{gross requirement}}{\text{DM intake}}$$

The absorption coefficient is the amount of a mineral absorbed by the animal through normal digestive pathways. It is comparable to the digestibility coefficients cited for fibre, protein, starch or other dietary components.

5.6.1 Major mineral nutrients

The major mineral nutrients that are considered in this section are calcium, phosphorus, magnesium, potassium, sodium, sulphur and chloride. The first three are considered in some detail, potassium, sodium and chloride will be considered together with the concept of dietary cation-anion balance (DCAB) and sulphur will be mentioned only in the context of protein metabolism.

5.6.1.1 Calcium

Calcium is one of the most common minerals in the cow. It is very important in maintaining a number of physiological and biochemical processes. Almost 99% of calcium is stored in hydroxyapatite in the inorganic matrix of the bone and teeth. The storage of calcium and the pattern and concentration of release of the element is the key to the animal's control of milk fever (hypopcalcaemia, parturient paresis). The role of calcium in milk fever will be considered in depth in Chapter 6. Calcium is also important for nerve function, contraction of muscles, blood clotting and a number of enzyme systems that drive the animal's metabolism. The efficiency of absorption of calcium and the degree with which it is utilised depends on the form of calcium supplied, the level and form of phosphorus and the supply of vitamin D. A ratio of Ca:P of 1:1 or 1:2 are appropriate for dairy cows.

The requirements for calcium for the dry cow have been examined in detail (unlike many minerals). The maintenance requirement is calculated from the endogenous loss of calcium in the faeces and that excreted in the urine. Even when the intake of calcium is very low, there is little reduction in the amount excreted and therefore correct supplementation during lactation is very important. The amount of calcium deposited during pregnancy is calculated in a similar fashion to energy and protein requirements, that is, the amount deposited in the amniotic fluid, membranes, foetus and the pregnant uterus (minus the normal levels in the non-pregnant uterus). Calcium from the diet has an absorption coefficient of approximately 68% in mature cows. The absorption coefficient for calcium in the sucking calf is approximately 95%. There are no data published for growing heifers.

Table 5.7 Net requirement for calcium in pregnant cows

Process	Requirement
Maintenance	16 mg Ca/kg live-weight
Pregnancy	
30 weeks	4.5 g Ca/day
35 weeks	8.2 g Ca/day
40 weeks	13.9 g Ca/day
Growth	14 g Ca/kg live-weight gain

Compiled from ARC (1980); NZAP (1983); NRC (1989)

The requirement for growth is relatively high in relation to the pregnancy requirement (Table 5.7). It is probably unwise to increase the level of calcium in the ration of a heifer to cover her requirements for growth during the last eight weeks of gestation even though milk fever is almost never observed in the primiparous cow.

5.6.1.2 Phosphorus

The function of phosphorus in the cow is to form hydroxyapatite in the bone matrix, to be incorporated into many important chemicals in the body for instance, phospholipids (cell membranes and the myelin sheath of the nervous system), adenosine triphosphate (ATP; the chemical that provides the cell its energy and drives many important metabolic pathways) and cyclic adenosine 3' 5'-monophosphate (cAMP; an important chemical implicated in the hormonal control of metabolism and physiology). Phosphorus metabolism, as mentioned, is interrelated with calcium metabolism. The major site of absorption is the small intestine (the same as Ca) and its uptake is stimulated by vitamin D. The uptake of P is thought to be controlled by formation of a metabolite of vitamin D (1,25 dihydroxycholecalciferol) in the kidney. Increases in the concentration of this metabolite in the gut mucosal cells enhance the absorption of P. The uptake of P is also affected by the level of calcium in the diet. Diets with a high ratio of Ca:P tend to lead to a lower absorption of P. Normally, if the ration is adequate in vitamin D a ratio of Ca:P of 1:1 or 1:2 will suffice. The majority of P is passed in the faeces with very little being excreted via the urine.

The requirements of P for maintenance, pregnancy and growth in cows are given in Table 5.8. The absorption coefficient used in mature cows is 0.58 but in young cattle the coefficient can be as high as 0.78.

In monogastric animals (pigs and poultry), the level of P in the diet is limited by complex organic molecules called phytates. Phytate P is unavailable to their digestion or metabolism but the presence of bacteria in the rumen with the correct enzymes will allow the utilisation of these chemicals.

Table 5.8 Net requirements for phosphorus (P) in pregnant cows

Process	Requirement
Maintenance	12 mg P/kg live weight
Pregnancy	
30 weeks	3.3 g/day
35 weeks	5.8 g/day
40 weeks	9.6 g/day
Growth	8 g/kg live-weight gain

Compiled from ARC (1980); NZAP (1983); NRC (1989)

5.6.1.3 Magnesium

Magnesium is an important element in the internal chemical reactions of the cell. It is a co-factor to many of the molecular changes mediated by enzymes in energy metabolism and it plays an important role in nerve impulse conduction and hence the processes of neural transmission (at the myoneural junction). Magnesium also has a function in the method of transfer of sodium and potassium across cell membranes (the Na-K activated Mg-ATPase pump), thus controlling the overall electrochemical gradient. About 70% of the total amount of magnesium in the cow is stored in bone but unlike Ca and P, it is unavailable to the cow. Only about 2% of the total amount of magnesium in the cow is available in the circulatory system at one time with the rest in the soft tissue (mainly the muscle). The amount of magnesium absorbed from the diet varies from 10 to 25% with a median of 17% for cows. The main factors which affect its absorption in the intestine are high levels of dietary potassium (decreases the absorption), as do some organic acids and protein (especially non-protein nitrogen). The requirements for magnesium are in Table 5.9.

Table 5.9 Net magnesium requirements for the cow in late pregnancy

Maintenance	3 mg/kg live weight
Pregnancy	
30 weeks	1.6 g/day
35 weeks	2.9 g/day
40 weeks	5.0 g/day
Growth	0.45 g/kg live-weight gain

Compiled from ARC (1980); NZAP (1983); NRC (1989)

Supplying magnesium in late pregnancy and early lactation is very important to ensure the cow does not suffer from the metabolic disorder of hypomagnesaemia (grass tetany).

5.6.1.4 Potassium, sodium and chloride

It is important to attempt to control the intake of potassium in the dry cow as excessive intake of the essential element is likely to depress the absorption of magnesium and hence leave the cow potentially prone to an increased risk of hypomagnesaemia. Potassium is essential to mammalian physiology as it is implicit in the control of acid-base metabolism, electrolyte and water balance and renal function. It is also essential for neural activity and muscle function (along with calcium controlling contraction). A cow in late pregnancy requires about 55 g/day. The majority of rations fed to dry cows will provide an excess of potassium and deficiency is unlikely to ever occur.

Sodium is essential in the maintenance of plasma osmolarity and hence the function of the red blood cell. It is involved in neural activity and the transfer of glucose across cell membranes (Na-K activated Mg-ATPase pump system). Estimated requirements for sodium for pregnant cows are in Table 5.10. The likelihood of sodium deficiency occurring is negligible if there is free access to a salt lick.

Table 5.10 Requirements for sodium in pregnancy

Maintenance	6.4 mg/kg live weight
Pregnancy (last 6 weeks)	2.2 g/day
Growth	1.6 g/kg live-weight gain

The absorption coefficient for sodium is 91%.

Compiled from ARC (1980); NZAP (1983); NRC (1989)

Chloride deficiency is unlikely to occur in ruminant livestock given normal diets. Chloride is the most important dietary anion (sulphate is the other) and it plays a role in the control of the electrolyte balance of plasma and cerebrospinal fluid.

5.6.1.5 Sulphur

Sulphur is essential for protein synthesis in all mammalian and bacterial systems and therefore the metabolism of the element is interrelated with nitrogen metabolism. Sulphur is also an important component in cartilage and tendons (in the form of chondroitin sulphate), in the blood as the anti-clotting factor heparin and in vitamins (especially the B complex, thiamine and biotin). Sulphur can occur in feeds in two forms; as inorganic sulphate and organic S compounds (for example amino acids e.g. methionine). The animal has a mechanism to ensure S is used efficiently and any lost to metabolism can be recycled via the saliva. The requirements of the cow in pregnancy have not been calculated but the diet must contain at least 1.3 to 1.8 g S/kg DM. With the reduction in S emissions from power stations and factories in the United Kingdom, the concentration of S in forages conserved for winter feeding has declined and in some regions sulphur is now necessary as part of the fertiliser top-dressing of grassland pastures.

5.6.2 Dietary Cation/Anion Balance (DCAB)

The balance of cations and anions ingested in the ration and water of a ruminant determines the acid-base metabolism of the body fluids. The net acidity ingested is the difference between the anions and cations consumed in the diet. It therefore follows that the net acidity output is the difference between the anions and cations excreted. The results of metabolism is the production of protons (H^+) and this component of the balance must be incorporated into the calculations of DCAB. In theory, DCAB is

$$(\text{Anion-Cation})_{in} + H^+ \text{ endogenous} - (\text{Anion-Cation})_{out} = 0$$

Another important theoretical consideration is;

[(sodium + potassium) - (chloride + sulphate)] / 100 g DM

where the concentrations of each element are represented as milliequivalents (meq).

The easiest method of calculating the DCAB of a diet is to use the following equation:

DCAB (meq/kgDM)=[(Na/0.229)+(K/0.39)]-[(Cl/0.3545)+(S/0.16)]

where Na, K, Cl and S are expressed as g/kg DM.

It is suggested that the optimal DCAB for diets offered in the dry period lies between +62 and -128 meq [(Na+K)-(Cl+S)]/kg DM. These diets are quite low in DCAB and therefore it is suggested that the lower the DCAB, the lower the potential risk of milk fever.

Dietary cation-anion difference may have a major impact on the physiology of the cow during pregnancy and lactation. The main effect of DCAB on the cow's physiology is concerned with the acid-base balance in the blood. The control of the blood's acid-base balance is centred on the kidney and its ability to excrete or retain certain minerals. If the DCAB is negative, an anionic diet (say -25 meq./100 g DM), slight metabolic acidosis occurs, whereas slight metabolic alkalosis occurs when the DCAB of the diet is positive.

Alleviation of hypocalcaemia in early lactation by nutritional manipulation of the ration in late pregnacy is highly effective. DCAB has been implicated as one possible mechanism. Diets with a negative DCAB may increase the efficiency of uptake of calcium in the intestine or an increase the rate of re-absorption of calcium into the skeleton (as a result of an increase in the activity of parathyroid hormone). However anionic diets must not be offered for extended periods as it will lead to an artificial manipulation of the systemic acid-base balance and may lead metabolic acidosis, increase the risk of osteoporotic conditions (fractures in old cows) and a change in the hormonal control of calcium mobilisation from the skeleton (calcitonin).

Research in the United States of America showed that serum calcium and phosphorus concentrations were elevated if cows in the dry period were offered diets with a negative DCAB (-25 meq./100 g DM) compared with a control diet (+5 meq./100 g DM). The incidence of hypocalcaemia was reduced by 50% in cows given a diets which had a negative DCAB.

Finally, many nutritionists do not as a matter of course ensure diets are assessed for concentration of Na, K, S and Cl. If DCAB is to be used as a management process for dry cows, these analysis are essential for accurate formulation of a ration. It is therefore very important to monitor voluntary DM intake during late pregnancy, especially the "close-up" period. Failure to eat adequate levels of feed can lead to a significant reduction in mineral intake and supplementation may be required. Supplementation of the ration with anionic salts may pose problems as a result of their variable palatability. Chloride salts tend to be more unpalatable than sulphate salts. Intake of water is another important variable to consider. Little research has been performed to assess the level of water required by the pregnant cow and therefore little is known about the interaction between mineralogical quality of water and intake by pregnant animals. It is also suggested that anionic salts should be offered for at least two weeks prior to calving and for no more than 4 weeks in total.

5.6.3 Trace elements

Eight trace elements are considered as essential for ruminant livestock. This section considers, in varying degrees of detail, iron, copper, zinc, manganese, cobalt, molybdenum, selenium and iodine.

5.6.3.1 Iron

The iron status of the cow in late pregnancy has to be considered in some detail. The reliance of the developing calf on its mother for the supply of oxygen and the removal of carbon dioxide is controlled by the presence of haemoglobin and carbonic anhydrase. The active centre of haemoglobin is elemental iron. Up to 65% of the iron stored in the cow is in haemoglobin (the rest is in other important haem-containing compounds, for example cytochrome, in pigments and enzymes). Ferritin, the transition iron storage protein, is found in the liver, spleen and bone marrow. Low concentrations are observed in milk and the presence of lactoferrin in milk ensures the levels of free iron are very low (see Chapter 4). The recommended concentration of iron in the diet of the dry cow is 40 mg/kg DM.

5.6.3.2 Copper and molybdenum

Copper has several functions in the metabolism of the cow. Copper is present in the blood plasma mainly (up to 80% of total) as ceruloplasmin. This ferroxidase is required to oxidise the ferrous (Fe (II)) ion to the ferric (Fe(III)) form thus allowing the mobilisation of iron from transferritin (in plasma) to ferretin (in tissues). Copper is necessary for the conversion of tyrosine to melanin (a reaction catalysed by the enzyme system polyphenyl oxidase). Therefore if copper is not adequately supplied via the ration, a lightening of the animals coat occurs mainly around the eyes (or other areas) leading to a "spectacled" appearance. Skeletal abnormalities can occur in new-born calves, probably as a result of a reduction in the number of cross-linkages in the bone matrix. The main problem seems to be an inadequate formation of collagen caused by low activity of the copper containing enzyme, lysyl oxidase.

The absorption of copper varies with age and dietary factors. Older animals tend to have a lower efficiency of absorption. In cattle the absorption coefficient can be as low as 0.05. Molybdenum, sulphur and iron all affect the uptake and utilisation of copper. With increasing concentration of Mo, S and Fe in the diet, the copper can be incorporated into compounds such as Cu-thiomolybdate. The majority of research into the formation of insoluble copper compounds in rumen has been performed on cows grazing the high Mo "teart pastures" in Somerset. The relationship between pasture Mo and copper adequacy is outlined in Table 5.11. It can be seen that a ratio of Cu:Mo of less than 2:1 results in potential copper deficiency. The requirements for copper in pregnant cows are shown in Table 5.12.

Molybdenum, although interacting strongly with copper, is essential in several enzyme systems in the cow. It is the active centre of xanthine oxidase, an important enzyme in the breakdown of nucleic acids. It also plays an important role in the reduction of the ferric, Fe (III) ion to enable it to be incorporated, as the ferrous ion, into ferritin. Increasing the concentration of sulphur seems to decrease the uptake of molybdenum in intestine. The level of Mo required by the cow seems to be very low, but how little is not yet known. Diets containing up to 2 mg Mo/kg DM seem to be adequate. Concentrations greater than this may well be a problem in copper metabolism.

Table 5.11 Relationship between Cu and Mo levels in pasture

Pasture level (mg/kg DM)

Mo	Cu	Ratio Cu: Mo	Notes
<2	3	>1.5:1	simple Cu deficiency
2	9	4.5:1	Cu adequate
5	9	1.8:1	Excessive Mo and Cu is inadequate
5	12	2.4:1	Mo not in excess and Cu adequate
7	12	1.7:1	Excessive Mo and Cu is inadequate
7	18	2.6:1	Mo not in excess and Cu adequate

Compiled from NZAP (1983)

Table 5.12 Requirements for copper in pregnant cows

Maintenance	7.1 μg/kg live weight
Pregnancy (last eight weeks)	2.07 mg Cu/day
Growth	1.0 mg Cu/kg live-weight gain

Compiled from ARC (1980); NZAP (1983); NRC (1989)

5.6.3.3 Zinc, Cobalt and Manganese

Zinc, manganese and cobalt are three essential trace elements required for the maintenance of various metabolic functions in the pregnant cow. Zinc is utilised as the active site of many metalloenzymes (e.g. carbonic anhydrase) that are essential for energy production and carbohydrate utilisation. It is also important in the synthesis of nucleic acids. As the ruminant has no long-term storage mechanism for zinc the requirement of the animal is fulfilled by a relatively constant supply via the diet or water. Failure to provide an adequate supply of zinc can lead to impaired reproductive performance, deterioration of hair, horn, skin (parakeratosis) and joints.

At parturition the concentration of zinc in the sera declines but will return to relatively normal values about 3 to 5 days post parturition. Cattle suffering from dystocia show a greater decline in the concentration of zinc in the blood sera immediately post parturition and the period to recovery after calving is extended. It has been shown that treatment of multiparous cows before calving with zinc is not effective against dystocia, however there are some preliminary reports that the use of zinc before calving in heifers may reduce the incidence of dystocia. The requirements for zinc are shown in Table 5.13.

Table 5.13 Requirements for zinc in pregnant cows

Pregnancy (last eight weeks)	1.1 to 6.3 mg Zn/day
Growth	24 mg Zn/kg live-weight gain

Compiled from ARC (1980); NZAP (1983); NRC (1989)

Cobalt is essential for the synthesis of vitamin B12 in the rumen. If inadequate vitamin B12 is synthesised the main effect on the metabolism of the cow is a block on the utilisation of propionate and therefore impaired energy metabolism. The symptoms of deficiency are impaired growth, anaemia and potential reduction in reproductive performance. Various methods of alleviation are available, for example pasture treatment, slow release boluses and feed blocks/licks.

Manganese is an important trace element implicated in various processes which affect pregnancy and development of a viable calf. Manganese is important in the synthesis of mucopolysaccharides in bone and teeth matrices, the synthesis of cholesterol, gluconeogenesis (especially the conversion of amino acids to energy yielding substrates) and in glucose utilisation. The diet should contain no less than 20 to 25 mg/kg DM and if lower concentrations are observed poor reproductive performance is noted as a result of delayed or irregular oestrus activity.

5.6.3.4 Selenium and Iodine

Selenium and iodine are important metalloid elements essential in tissue metabolism and hormonal control of metabolic processes. Selenium is important in the synthesis of glutathione peroxidase (GSP-Px) which reduces the impact of peroxides in metabolism. Selenium in conjunction with vitamin E are therefore important in the prevention of oxidative damage to all cellular and tissue types. The classical symptom of selenium deficiency is white muscle disease in calves.

Iodine is important in the formation of thyroid hormones. It is therefore essential for the development of the foetus, especially the development of the brain, heart and lung. Iodine is also implicated in lung maturation in the foetus. Typical signs of deficiency are classified by goitre or reduction in foetal weight or viability. Both iodine and selenium supplementation can occur through mineral supplementation, feed blocks, licks and injection (in the case of selenium).

5.7 Live-weight gain and foetal growth - a paradox

It has been mentioned in an earlier section, that weighing cattle is difficult on farm. The two methods available are the calibrated weigh crush or the weigh-band. The use of a weigh-band is relatively simple and unlikely to be affected by the stage of pregnancy. Simply use the band according to the manufacturer's directions which generally suggest the band is used around the heart-girth of the cow.

During late pregnancy, the cow herself can gain weight at 0.3 to 0.5 kg/day (as well as lose weight in certain conditions), although an overall live-weight change of between 0.5 and 1.0 kg/day can be observed in late pregnancy. What is the contribution to live-weight gain of the foetus and is the cow herself increasing or decreasing her own body weight? This is one of the most important questions to be answered when considering the construction of a ration for the dry period.

The calculation for energy and protein requirement in pregnancy can be modified to consider the situation outlined above. Foetal growth during the last 8 weeks of pregnancy seems to be relatively constant, with no decline in the very last days of pregnancy. The typical gains in weight of the foetus plus pregnant uterus during pregnancy are outlined in Table 5.14.

Table 5.14 Daily gain in live-weight of foetus plus pregnant uterus during pregnancy.

Weeks	20	24	28	32	36	40
Live-weight gain (kg/day)	0.19	0.27	0.37	0.48	0.60	0.72

By difference, the change in live-weight of the cow herself can be calculated and therefore the requirements for energy, protein and minerals for the dam could be adjusted. In practice, many farmers attempt to achieve zero weight change during the dry period, however this approach must be questioned as the foetus is growing rapidly. Therefore if zero weight gain is achieved, and the foetus is growing, the dam must be losing some weight.

5.8 The question of twins and how to adjust the ration

It is considered that the combined weight of twins is generally 1.75 times the weight of a single calf. The level of energy and protein can probably be adjusted safely to ensure adequate supply to the developing calves, but it is not as clear cut for the mineral allowance.

5.9 Condition scoring

The condition score of the cow at calving reflects a number of factors which may or may not be interdependent. For instance the condition of the cow is related to the level of energy offered in diet, the requirement of the cow for energy, the intake of the ration and the condition score of the animal as she enters the dry period. It is therefore very important to ensure the condition score of the cow is monitored throughout late lactation and late pregnancy as it is potentially easier (and less risky) to alter the ration in late lactation than in the final stages of the dry period. It is more efficient to replace tissue energy stores during late lactation than in the dry period. If over-conditioning of the cow occurs during late lactation, yield of milk and animal health during the first 6 weeks of lactation may be compromised.

Various condition scoring systems have been used in different parts of the world. The system usually used in Great Britain has six scores ranging from 0 to 5. The scores are also sub-divided into halves. In the United States of America and New Zealand, a ten point scale is used. In Great Britain, the body condition score takes into consideration the level of fat and muscle cover over the spinous processes of the lumbar vertebrae, the fat cover of the transverse processes and the transition between the transverse process and the para-lumbar fossa. Also the fat and muscle cover of the tail-head (sacral vertebrae, hock and pin bones) and between the hock and pin bones are assessed.

The aim of the scores is to allow an indication to be given of the state of fatness or thinness of the individual cow and the status of the herd. While the system is relatively subjective, it is reasonably consistent for individual herdsmen scoring cattle. Even though the system has been criticised for its subjectivity, it has been shown by many researchers to have a strong correlation with body fat content. Therefore one of the major advantages of the system is that it can indicate how individual animals are faring in their weight loss or gain. It is estimated that a change in one unit of condition score is equivalent to about 80 kg of live-weight. Other estimates have suggested the change in a unit of condition score is equivalent to 50 to 60 kg of live weight. However these changes in weight depend on breed and individual type of animal and stage of production. The use of a weigh-band in conjunction with condition scoring is an important practical method to monitoring the ration being offered to ensure it is adequate in its formulation.

Condition scoring by palpation only assesses the sub-cutaneous cover of fat (the fat directly under the skin) but cows store fat in other parts of their bodies. Research has shown that although condition score may change, the proportion of fat stored in each of the major internal deposits varies little. The distribution of fat in the cow during late pregnancy is about 35 to 40% in or related to the muscle (intra and inter-muscular fat), 25 to 30% in the abdomen (especially near to the kidney) and about 14 to 18% directly under the skin (sub-cutaneous fat).

Cows should be scored, if possible, every two weeks and their scores mapped and compared with the targets set for the herd at the various stages of the production cycle. The main points in the scoring system are listed below:

Condition Score 0 The spines of the backbone are very prominent and there is no fat cover over the transverse processes or between para lumbar processes of the back. The tailhead appears raised and the ribs are very prominent. Under the tail a very deep cavity or depression with all the bones able to be felt, the skin very taught over the bones and each tail bone visible and the edges sharp. On palpation, the skin is drawn tight over the pelvis. Condition scores of zero are thankfully very rare in the United Kingdom as they indicate not just malnutrition but starvation or some chronic disease of the animal.

Condition Score 1 The spines of the backbone are still very prominent; the transverse processes very easy to feel but no longer sharp. The tailhead is still prominent and the ribs still project. Under the tail a deep depression with all the bones easily felt, the skin taught over the bones and the tail bones each clearly visible. The cow is emaciated.

Condition Score 2 The spines of the backbone can still be felt but are less prominent; the transverse processes can still be felt but there is some material present between them and the skin. The tailhead is no longer prominent and the individual ribs may not be visible. Under the tail a depression with a little fat present but the bones can still be easily felt, but individual tail bones are not visible and covered with tissue. The cow is in moderate condition for lactation but too thin for late pregnancy.

Condition Score 3 The spines of the backbone are still palpable with the transverse processes can only be felt by placing pressure over them. The ribs can only be detected by feeling them. Under the tail there is a shallow depression with some fat present but the pelvic bones can still be felt with some pressure, but with the individual tail bones not visible and covered with tissue. The condition of the cow is probably right for an animal in late pregnancy. For a cow in lactation, the condition is good.

Condition Score 4 There is muscle and fat above the spines of the backbone and they may just about be felt; the transverse processes cannot be felt even with firm pressure. The ribs cannot be felt. Under the tail there is a very slight depression with fat present although the pelvic bones can be felt with difficulty and the tail bones are not visible and covered with tissue. The cow is fat and at her maximum condition for late pregnancy.

Condition Score 5 There is much fat over the spines of the backbone; the transverse processes are covered by an obvious layer of fat. The ribs are covered by an obvious layer of fat. Under the tail there are folds of fat and the pelvic bones are difficult to feel or cannot be felt and the tail bones are not visible and covered with tissue. The cow is obese and suffers from severe over-conditioning. **It should be pointed out here that it is very difficult, and may compromise the health and welfare of the cow, to "slim" an over-conditioned cow. The process should not be attempted unless under strict veterinary supervision.**

It is recommended that cows should calve down at a condition score of 3.0 to 3.5 and the change in condition score in late pregnancy should not be excessive (a maximum of 1.0 unit in the last 8 weeks of pregnancy). Therefore the target condition score at drying-off should be about 2.5 to 3.0. Condition scores of greater than 3.0 to 3.5 do not benefit production of milk during the following lactation and may well impair milk production (See Chapter 6).

5.10 Historical development of dry cow rations

The rations fed to dry cows have changed considerably over the last 40 years. It is important to consider what developments have occurred in rationing of dry cows to gain a greater understanding of the philosophy of feeding the dry cow.

5.10.1 Pre 1940

During the majority of the 20th Century the feeding and rationing of dry cows received little attention by nutritionists or veterinarians. The majority of rationed offered to cows in late pregnancy were slight deviations from those used as production rations. Typically a simple formulation was based on maintenance plus 9 litres (2 gallons). A rations such as that would allow, at term, sufficient energy and protein for the cow and the calf. However in the early part of the dry period, the ration would provided a substantial surplus in energy and the cow would put on body weight and condition rapidly. Rations were formulated on roughages such as hay, straw, silage, turnips and mangolds with concentrate feeds of linseed, cotton meal, bran or palm kernel.

In modern feeding standards, the ration would supply about 100 MJ of metabolisable energy per day and 1034 g crude protein per day. A cow weighing 600 kg live weight and in her last 14 days of pregnancy, she would have a metabolisable energy requirement of approximately 100 MJ/day and require 510 g metabolisable protein per day. The formation of microbial protein is limited by a lack of eRDP in the ration (730 g eRDP), however the deficit is rectified by the supply of digestible but undegradable protein (150 g DUP). In theory the ration is sufficient in metabolisable energy and metabolisable protein (a surplus of about 110 g MP per day). It would however be unlikely that the cow would ingest the complete ration as about 60% of the ration is straw.

A typical ration for dry cows fed at the turn of the century was

Linseed cake	0.4 kg DM/day
Decorticated cotton cake	0.4 kg DM/day
Straw	7.0 kg DM/day
Turnips	4.0 kg DM/day

Source: McConnell, 1906.

5.10.2 1940 to 1980

An important development in the strategies of rationing and feeding the dry cow occurred during the late 1940s and early 1950s. Professor Boutflour developed a sophisticated system of dry cow feeding which, with some modification, is still in use today. The system was based on the premise that if a cow was "fit for the vigours of milk production", feeding the cow a correctly formulated ration during the dry period was essential. This opinion is now taken for granted and universally accepted. Over-feeding of cows, using the maintenance plus system, lead inevitably to a rapid deposition of condition and resulted in animals which suffered from inappetence in early lactation. Boutflour also observed that the cow in ideal condition could not eat enough feed during the first four to six weeks of lactation to sustain an increasing level of milk production and therefore her body weight and condition rapidly declined.

The process of "steaming-up" would begin about six to eight weeks before calving, almost immediately after drying-off. It was suggested that the dry cow should be brought into the buildings where she would be housed throughout the subsequent lactation and the parlour to "orientate her to her surroundings". This approach to management of the dry cow may not be a good idea as the stimulation of being taken into the parlour may extend the processes of lactogenesis and lead to a slowing in the rate of involution of the udder.

The ration to be fed during the "steaming-up" period should consist of a concentrate-based feed and the level of feeding being decided on the basis of cow condition and potential yield. Cows were generally grouped according to potential yield. The grouping of cows of high, medium and low yield potential can be difficult especially if there is limited space to house the animals. It has been suggested in previous chapters that dry cows should be housed in straw yards rather than cubicles to reduce the incidence of disease in the dry period and remove the likelihood of the cow injuring herself during calving. It is possible to modify straw yard systems (if space allows) to ensure groups of cows of different yield potential or condition score can be housed and fed different rations.

The recommended practice of "steaming-up" was to feed the cow between 0.5 and 2.5 kg of concentrate DM (about 0.7 to 3.0 kg fresh-weight) per head at six weeks prior to calving. The level of feeding was set by the condition of the cow entering the dry period. Lean animals (probably cows of condition score less than 2.5) were fed 2.5 kg of concentrate DM daily , cows of good condition (say a score between 2.5 to 3.5) were offered 1.5 kg DM of concentrate (about 1.75 kg of fresh-weight) per day and cows with excessive condition (approximately 3.5 to 4.5) were given 0.5 kg DM (about 0.7 kg fresh-weight) daily. A roughage (for example hay, silage or kale) was offered *ad libitum.* The principle of substitution of forage by concentrate would then play a role in the future pattern of feeding. This was however not always the case and cows with high condition scored (greater than 4) at calving resulted. Steaming up to ensure an increase of condition score of one unit during the dry period was reported to have a positive effect on milk yield and it was suggested that cows with a condition score of 2 or less would not reach potential milk yield.

The feeding of concentrate was increased by about 0.5 to 1.0 kg of concentrate DM per week from six weeks before calving to one week before calving. A further complexity was added to take into account the potential yield of the cow in the next lactation. The table below (Table 5.15) outlines the level of feeding of concentrates in the last week of pregnancy of cows expected to give different levels of milk production at peak lactation.

Table 5.15 Recommended level of feeding (kg DM/day) of cows of different condition score and expected level of production.

Condition score at drying-off	Expected milk yield at peak lactation (litres/day)					
	22	27	31	36	39	44
	Concentrates (kg DM/day)					
<2.5	4.5	5.5	6.5	7.5	8.5	9.0
2.5 - 3.5	3.5	4.5	5.5	6.5	7.5	8.5
3.5 +	2.5	3.5	4.5	5.5	6.5	7.5

Source: Russell (1969)

The system applied for heifers (or cattle of unknown milking ability) would not allow the level of concentrate feeding to be greater than 2.5 kg DM/day in the last week of pregnancy.

One of the most important issues to be discussed in detail is the type of concentrate offered during the dry period. Table 5.16 shows the level of concentrate DM that Professor Boutflour recommended for the dry cow. Boutflour performed his work using palm kernel meal; a feed which has a moderate energy density (11.1 MJ/kg DM) and moderate to high levels of undegradable but digestible protein (DUP). Palm kernel meal also contains high levels of cell walls and therefore makes it a feed with moderate to low palatability.

Table 5.16 Quantities of feed recommended for pregnant dry cows according to body condition score and potential milk yield

Condition Score	Yield potential	Hay intake (kg)	Palm Kernel Meal (kg)	Balances ME	eRDP	DUP
2.5	Low	5.5	4.5	12	-58	+465
3.5	Low	7.5	2.5	-20	-94	+359
2.5	High	1.0	9.0	+8	+28	+635
3.5	High	2.5	7.5	+0	-5	+572

Recalculated from Russell (1969) using AFRC (1993).

If we consider the rations developed by Boutflour using current feeding standards, the balances for metabolisable energy, eRDP and DUP can be calculated for the 600 kg cow in the last week of pregnancy, neither gaining or losing live-weight. We must also consider that the diets would have been offered with a medium quality hay.

If dry cows are kept at grass, grazing must be judged on its milk production value. Early spring grass in plentiful supply was estimated to be equivalent to 7.0 kg DM of concentrate used for steaming-up. Dependent on the condition and the estimated productivity of the cow, low levels or no supplementation of grazing would be necessary in early spring. When the quality of the grazing had declined (mid to late summer) or the grass was restricted in some way, concentrate supplementation at grass was deemed necessary for the dry cow. If the grass was of low digestibility but plentiful, concentrates were used to steam the cow up but grazing was restricted to ensure the cows had the appetite for the concentrate ration.

In the United States of America, rations used to "steam-up cows" were generally based on at least one-third of the roughage as alfalfa (lucerne) hay and a mixture of grain+concentrate. Typically, if the ration contained legume hay, the crude protein content of the grain concentrate component of the ration was approximately 12% in the dry matter, but if no legume hay was used the grain ration protein content was increased to at least 16% in the DM. Two common grain rations which were offered in the dry period are shown in Table 5.17.

Table 5.17 Typical concentrate rations for dry cows in the United States in the 1940s to 1950s.

Ration 1 Offered to cows given a roughage diet ad libitum which contained one-third of total roughage DM as alfalfa hay.

Concentrate	**% in total ration**
Ground maize	38
Ground oats	30
Wheat bran	25
Linseed meal	5
Bone-meal	1
Salt (NaCl)	1

Ration 2 Offered to cows given roughage containing little or no alfalfa hay.

Concentrate	**% in ration**
Ground maize	29.5
Ground oats	25
Wheat bran	25
Linseed meal	18
Bone-meal	1
Ground limestone	0.5
Salt (NaCl)	1

Source: Morrison (1949)

If the cow was in fairly good condition entering the dry period, she would be offered about 1 to 2 kg DM of the grain mixture daily with access to a high quality roughage ad libitum (hay, alfalfa hay or maize silage). If however the cow was not in good condition, she could receive up to 2 to 3 kg DM per day or more. Using the grain rations it was suggested that no more than 5.0 kg DM was to be given per day as it would be uneconomical and lead to cows with a low appetite in early lactation (fat-cow syndrome).

If the cows were kept at pasture and grass was plentiful, no supplementation with concentrates occurred; a system identical to that described above for the United Kingdom. Likewise, if the grazing was poor, cattle were supplemented with concentrates to ensure the cows maintained condition.

Another method of ensuring cows were in adequate condition for milk production was developed in Tennessee in the mid 1940s. This method was based on the use of concentrates to increase the condition of the cow during late lactation and feeding the dry cows a roughage (albeit of high quality) ration without concentrates through the dry period. This method would use the same amount of concentrates as the "traditional" method but it was suggested that it resulted in fewer cases of dystokia.

5.10.3 Post 1980

It has been realised in the last 20 years that the nutrition of the dry cow is as complex as the nutrition of the lactating cow. The method of rationing should be subdivided into two main sections according to the changes in the physiology of the cow. As mentioned at the outset of this Chapter the two sections of the dry period are from 56 days to 21 days prior to calving (the so-called "far-off dry period") and from 21 days to calving (the "close-up dry period").

5.10.3.1 Energy density of the ration

In general energy density of the ration is increased during the dry period to conpensate for the decline in voluntary feed intake of the cow. The exception to this rule is the inclusion of fat to the diet.

Dietary fat typically contains 35 MJ/kg DM and therefore their use in the "close-up dry period" is attractive to counter the decline in voluntary intake and hence decline in energy intake. It is important to note that inclusions of fat of greater than 5% in the total ration can affect the fermentation of other feeds in the rumen by "coating" feed particles and reducing their breakdown. Diets which contain high levels of fat have been implicated with inappetence, ketosis, hypocalcaemia and hypomagnesaemia in early lactation. To counter the increased risk of hypocalcaemia, it may be necessary to increase the calcium concentration of the lactation diet by 0.1% in the dry matter.

It has been suggested that an increase in energy density of the diet during the dry period will increase the concentration of protein in the milk during the subsequent lactation. However this response is not universally accepted. The major problem of increasing the energy density of the diet in late pregnancy is the rapid increase in body condition. If however the cow become too fat as a result of over feeding energy in late pregnancy, inappetence and other metabolic disorders may occur (see Chapter 6 for a more in depth discussion).

Manipulation of energy density in late pregnancy has lead to variable responses in the subsequent lactation. Researchers in the USA found that increasing the energy density of the diet in the "close-up dry period" increased both voluntary intake and milk yield in the subsequent lactation. Other researchers observed the contrary. In the United Kingdom, the current philosophy on feeding of energy in the "far-off dry period" is to maintain live-weight and body condition (that is to feed to the requirements of maintenance and pregnancy) in cattle with good condition (between 3.0 and 3.5). Lead feeding, the feeding of the production ration during the "close-up dry period", is necessary to adapt the rumen microflora to the type of ration given in lactation as well as attempting to increase voluntary intake. This strategy will have little effect on the overall condition of the cow or her live-weight as the decline in voluntary intake by the cow is offset by the increase in energy content of the ration. Care must however be taken when formulating the diet for mineral requirement (especially calcium).

5.10.3.2 Protein feeding

It is interesting to note that the requirement for protein calculated for pregnancy come from a series of data which are nearly 40 years old. Formulation of a ration adequate in crude protein with a composition of the protein meeting the demands of the rumen microflora and the intermediary metabolism of the cow is difficult. Furthermore the interaction between the dietary supply of protein and mobilisation of maternal protein reserves had to be considered carefully.

Much of the crude protein given in the diet is converted in the rumen to bacterial protein, amino acids and ammonia. Therefore the supply of protein from the diet must be in a form that ensures optimal microbial synthesis. Any factor that reduces the "availability" or reduces the net intake of protein during late pregnancy may well reduce foetal growth and development. Short term restriction in supply of protein to the foetus are more detrimental than restrictions in energy as the requirements of the foetus for amino acids as both precursors for tissue deposition and as a supply of energy have to be maintained. Manipulation of the maternal protein reserve is therefore essential to formulate a ration that does not supply too high levels of energy to the cow nor reduce the supply of amino acids and glucose to the developing calf. It is therefore suggested that cows in late pregnancy should be given an adequate (but not excessive supply, that is 5% above maintenance requirements for pregnancy) of dietary energy and high levels of digestible but undegradable protein.

As the cow has no specific mechanism to store surplus nitrogen it is generally cleared via urea metabolism and excretion. However during periods of shortage, the cow can mobilise protein from her body reserves (for example muscle). Protein catabolism and anabolism are essentially processes which provide a labile store of protein that can be used under periods of malnutrition or physiological stress (for example in late pregnancy or early lactation). These processes are however balanced finely by the rates of accretion and degradation in skeletal muscle tissue and linked to energy metabolism and possibly mediated by thyroid activity. The aim of the dry period should be to increase the labile protein store to an optimal level therefore providing a supply of amino acids for either direct synthesis of milk protein acting as an energy substrate in mammary gland metabolism.

A typical ration that will fulfill the requirements of the pregnant cow and ensure there is adequate "loading" to the maternal protein store is outlined below.

Grass silage supplying 80 MJ/day (7.3 kg DM/day)

High DUP concentrate (for example prairie meal or protected soya) providing 30 MJ/day (approximately 2.5 kg DM/day dependent on metabolisable energy content and feed type).

Total ME supply from the diet	110 MJ/day
eRDP supply	946 g/day
DUP supply	285 g/day

The ration is based on the supply of DUP under restricted supply of metabolisable energy. Diets such as the one shown have been shown to increase milk yield, the concentration of protein in the milk or both during the first 6 to 10 weeks of lactation. Whether the response is due to an increased supply of glucogenic substrates (energy yielding) or an increased flexibility in the cow's intermediary metabolism to draw on both labile energy and protein reserves have not been elucidated.

MCP is limited by energy and therefore 845 g protein is available for microbial protein synthesis yielding about 540 g MTP for the cow. If the cow's MP requirement is about 580 g/day, the requirement must be made up by DUP, of which there is a surplus in this diet. The cow therefore has the option to utilise the amino acid supply from microbial protein and DUP either to support pregnancy or to build maternal reserves. If the diet however had a significant surplus in eRDP, the cost of excretion of excess urea in metabolism has to be considered, which may utilise some of the amino acids supplied from DUP. Diets which do not contain a significant surplus in DUP, fail to supply adequate amino acids to allow the flexibility in metabolism.

5.9.3.3 Milk production response to feeding high levels of DUP during the dry period.

Manipulation of milk production during early lactation is normally brought about by changes in the level of supply of carbohydrate to the cow. This manipulation of the "glucogenic" status of the cow usually has the greatest impact on the production of milk casein (a milk protein important in cheese production). Normally the greatest response is in milk protein yield rather than increased milk protein concentration.

There is a degree of inconsistency of response of milk production to feeding high levels DUP in the diet of the expectant cow. Several studies in the United Kingdom have shown responses of between 0.05 and 0.3% increases in milk protein concentration and/or increases in milk yield of between 0 and 3.5 kg/day during early lactation. These studies are not simply cases of supplying more protein to the cows during the dry period, but supplying protein sources of the correct amino acid balance and modifying the supply to be utilised at different points in the digestive tract (i.e. the supply of DUP).

The mechanisms for the increase in milk yield and/or protein after supplementation with DUP are poorly understood. A possible theory to understand the process is the relative control of the labile stores of the maternal protein pool and the efficiency of utilisation of eRDP for MTP production. It is not known how much labile store is utilised as amino acid N and how much is lost to general circulation and therefore to catabolic processes. The latter point has implications in tissue energy metabolism. Any increase in milk yield is simply not a function of supply of nutrients, but has to be considered in light of any increases in secretory tissue mass. The response of increased production of secretory tissue in the mammary gland is mediated by increases in natural endogenous growth hormone. The carry-over effect into early lactation of increased production of growth hormone could lead to an increase in milk production.

Further recommended reading

AFRC (1993) *Energy and Protein Requirements of Ruminants.* An advisory manual prepared by the AFRC. Technical Committee on Responses to Nutrients CAB International, Wallingford, UK.

ARC (1980) *The Mineral Nutrition of Livestock.* CAB Slough, UK.

Bellows, R.A. and Short, R.E. (1978). Effects of precalving feed level on birth weight, calving difficulty and subsequent fertility. *Journal of Animal Science* **46**:1522.

Burhans, W.S. and Bell, A.W. (1997) Feeding the transition cow. *Proceedings of the Cornell Feed Manufacturers Conference.*

Carstons, G.E., Johnson, D.E., Holland, M.D. and Odde, K.G. (1987) Effects of prepartum protein nutrition and birthweight on basal metabolism in bovine neonates. *Journal of Animal Science* **65**: 745.

Curtis, C.R., Erb, H.N., Sniffen, C.J., Smith, R.D. and Kronfeld, D.S. (1985) Path analysis of dry period nutrition, post partum metabolic and reproductive disorders and mastitis in Holstein cows. *Journal of Dairy Science* **68**: 2347.

Grummer, R.R. (1995) Impact of changes in organic nutrient metabolism on feeding the transition dairy cow. *Journal of Animal Science* **73**: 2820.

Hayirli, A., Grummer, R.R., Nordheim, E., Crump, P., Beede, D.K., VandeHaar, M.J. and Kilmer, L.H. (1998) A mathematical model for describing dry matter intake of transition cows. *Journal of Dairy Science* **81**: 296.

Hidiroglou, M. and Knipfel, J.E. (1981) Maternal-Fetal relationships of copper, manganese and sulphur in ruminants. A review. *Journal of Dairy Science* **64**: 1637.

Hill, J. and Roberts, D.J. (1994) Effect of dry cow feeding on milk protein yield. *SAC Staff Note No. 78.*

McConnell, P (1906) *Agricultural Notebook.*

Morrison, F (1949) *Feeds and Feeding.* Morrison Publishing Ltd, Ithaca, USA.

National Research Council (1989) *Nutrient requirements of dairy cattle.* NRC, Washington DC. USA.

NZAP (1983) *The mineral requirements of grazing ruminants.* New Zealand Society of Animal Production.

Polan, C.E. and Fisher, R.J. (1993) Nutrition can affect concentration of milk protein. Feedstuffs June 14 1993.

Russell, K. (1969) *The Principles of Dairy Farming.* Farming Press, Ipswich, UK.

Van Saun, R.J., Idleman, S.C. and Sniffen, C.J. (1993) Effect of undegradable protein amount fed prepartum on post partum production in first lactation Holstein cows. *Journal of Dairy Science* **76**: 236.

Chapter 6

NUTRITIONAL AND METABOLIC DISORDERS

6.1 Introduction

Many nutritional and metabolic disorders that occur in early lactation have their basis in late pregnancy. The increased incidence of hypocalcaemia (milk fever) and retained placenta in older cows is a normal observation, even when the nutritional management of the animals is excellent. However if poor management of the cow occurs in late pregnancy a number of problems can occur. A greater incidence of retained placenta, as a result of poor management is likely to lead to an increase in metritis and chronic acetonaemia. If cows suffer from mild acetonaemia they may have an increased risk of left displaced abomasum which in turn may increase the risk of chronic acetonaemia. The aim of this chapter is to focus on the metabolic and nutritional problems in early lactation that are caused by poor nutritional management in the dry period.

6.2 The downer cow

This condition is generally seen in the period at or soon after calving and probably involves a large number of different entities. Most of these cases follow milk fever which has been treated successfully but the cow fails to rise. By definition a true downer cow is apparently perfectly normal and is eating and drinking well, dunging and urinating as usual but just does not get up. The types of problem which can be involved are listed in Table 6.1. This list is anything but exhaustive although it is still very long. In some cases if the animal partly rises and then looses her grip and slips she may loose confidence to try again.

Table 6.1 Some of the causes of "downer cow" syndrome

Metabolic	Toxaemia	Injuries during calving	Injuries following calving	Management	Miscellaneous
Milk fever	Coliform mastitis	Ruptured uterus	Fractured pelvis	Malnutrition	BSE
Magnesium deficiency	Staphylococcal mastitis	Internal haemorrhage	Fractured femur	Over-fat	Acidosis
	Streptococcus uberis (mastitis)				
Phosphorus deficiency	Toxic metritis	Obturator paralysis	Rupture of pelvic round ligament	Delayed calcium therapy	Bloat
Potassium deficiency	Acute diffuse peritonitis	Sacral displacement	Dislocated hip	Veterinary treatment (e.g. epidural)	Hypothermia
Displaced abomasum	Rupture of uterus, abomasum, reticulum.	Fractured pelvis	Ruptured upper hind leg muscles	Slippery floors	Heat stroke
Excess magnesium	Aspiration pneumonia	Exhaustion	Ruptured Achilles tendon		
Acetonaemia	Traumatic reticulitis, pericarditis		Damage to limb nerves		
Fat cow syndrome					
			Pressure syndrome following milk fever		

The main problem with all these animals is to know whether or not they are likely to get up. This is very difficult to decide but the longer they are down the worse the prognosis. Generally about half are up within four days with appropriate nursing. If an animal is down longer than about 10 to 14 days then it is unlikely to rise, although the odd animal has risen after a month.

Several factors can help to make the decision as to whether or not to persist with an individual animal. If the cow shows any new signs which increase or start while recumbent then it is unlikely to rise. Thus if the animal shows nervous signs of either excessive dullness or it is very excitable then there is likely to be due to brain involvement and it usually means a poor outcome. The positioning of the legs can also be significant and if the animal can slightly lift its weight and move forward, the so-called "creeper" or "crawler" then this is a good sign. If the animal appears "frog legged" with the hind legs partially bent and placed slightly behind the cow then this is usually a good sign. If the hind legs are extended forwards so that they are almost in contact with the elbows or they are placed out behind the body, then these are bad signs.

When the animal tends to rest on one side, and if she is then moved to the other side she returns to the first position then again the cow is less likely to rise than if she will rest on either side. If there is not the will to nurse these animals then their prognosis is poor. Indeed on many busy farms there is insufficient time to devote to cows which are down without neglecting the rest of the herd and in such cases it is in the best interests of the cow to arrange early slaughter.

Treatment should involve an early assessment by your veterinary surgeon of the cow and whether or not she is likely to rise. Regular visits should be made to determine whether or not progress or deterioration is occurring. Therapy will include rectifying any metabolic deficiencies such as calcium, phosphorus, magnesium and potassium. Anti-inflammatory agents can help where the underlying problem is one of damage whether nerve, muscle or bone (but obviously not fractures or dislocations). Stimulants and vitamin injections may be of use. Tonics may be helpful whether therapy is given and good nursing is essential.

The cow should have her legs massaged, worked and the cow must be turned from side to side. The number of times the cow is moved per day should be an odd number so that she does not remain on the same side each night. The use of inflatable bags or a support net or harness which can then be attached to the fore end loader to gently lift the cow and allow her legs to be worked and improve their circulation can be very helpful. Often a combination of a inflatable bag and some form of net or hoist is best as they support the cow from above and below. Warm water baths using a mobile swimming tank can be another method of helping maintain movement and leg circulation.

Good quality feed should be offered and must be accessible to the animal and the same with water. She will need to have the pressure relieved from her udder and checked for mastitis. Shade and shelter should be provided if outside and the cow should be protected from the others in the herd by keeping her on her own or placing barriers or a ring feeder around her. Indoors she must be well bedded on a floor surface which is not slippery and will give her some purchase if she attempts to rise. If a cow tries to rise and is uncertain of her footing, she may then refuse to try again. The doors of any box in which she is kept must open outwards.

6.3 Endometritis

This condition can occur soon after calving, particularly when it has been protracted and where there has been some manual assistance to the parturition. Poor hygiene at calving has also been implicated as has problems such as fatty liver and hypocalcaemia. In a normal animal the uterus has contracted to its normal non pregnant size by 35 days after calving. By five weeks 70% of cows will have had one oestrus and five to 10% two heats. Oestrus with its increased tension within the uterus and the further opening of the cervix helps to expel any uterine pus or other debris from the organ. Retained placentas also tend to increase the likelihood of the problem. Up to the time of first heat infection albeit at a low level can be detected in about 75% of cows. This first oestrus rapidly and dramatically reduces the number affected.

Endometritis is defined as an inflammation of the inner lining of the uterus, the endometrium. It is usually seen 21 days or more after calving and results in the presence of a uterine discharge which contains pus. This is usually yellow or brownish-red, and can be very liquid or more jelly-like and sometimes consists of only a few flecks of pus in clear gelatinous material. Sometimes it is rather smelly. The condition results in a delay in the uterus returning to its normal non pregnant size and probably occurs in about 10% of all calved cows. Obviously the problem is one of infection and as the uterus is thought to be sterile during normal pregnancy the organisms which are environmental in origin enter at or after calving. When an abortion occurs infection may occur during that process. There are a large number of factors which influence whether or not the problem arises. Some of the many causes of endometritis are given in Table 6.2.

Table 6.2 Some of the factors which can contribute to endometritis

Calving factors	Uterine factors	Cow/other factors	Nutritional factors
Dystocia	Bacterial flora	Breed	Fatty liver
Retained placenta	Uterine involution rate	Stress	Acetonaemia
Calving environment	Uterine defense mechanisms	Induction of parturition	Milk fever
Calving hygiene		Gestation length	Protein deficient diet
Calving assistance		Last lactation milk yield	Overfeeding in the dry period
Twins		Extended dry period	Selenium deficiency
Abortion		Season of year	Vitamin E deficiency
		Return to oestral activity	
		Number of calvings	
		Suckling	

The signs are usually of the presence of some purulent discharge which is usually seen at the vulva and on the tail of the cow. The problem has a detrimental effect on fertility with an increase in the calving to conception interval, more services to successful conception and an increased culling rate compared with normal unaffected cows. A large number of different forms of treatment are undertaken including antibiotics, hormones or various antiseptic solutions. There is considerable debate about treatment efficacy as most cattle will slowly overcome the problem with successive oestruses. The antibiotic can be given by injection or into the uterus in a pessary or an infusion. Intrauterine infusion by the veterinary surgeon of the antibiotic oxytetracycline can provide some improvement in the fertility of some cows.

Hormones used can include oestrogens which increase the resistance to infection and increase the uterine tone which with the opening of the cervix helps remove the pus within the uterus. Prostaglandins by injection help to increase oestrogen activity. The use of gonadotrophin releasing hormone (GnRH) and its analogues has been tried with variable success. Antiseptics have been inserted into the uterus including Lugol's iodine, other iodine solutions and chlorhexidine. Results have often been contradictory and in some instances fertility has been reduced.

6.4 Metabolic disorders

6.4.1 Milk Fever

This is a problem of calcium deficiency around the time of calving. The demand for calcium for milk production even in a moderately producing cow is usually about three times greater than for a pregnant animal. This sudden switch in demands means that in all cows there is a fall in blood calcium levels around calving. At this time there are three factors which have an important influence, namely excess loss of calcium in the colostrum, impairment in absorption of calcium from the intestines around calving and mobilisation of the calcium stores of the body is not sufficiently rapid. At the time of calving there is a natural decrease in feed uptake and the gut slows down thereby reducing overall absorption.

The problem of milk fever is common and, on average, up to 10% of cows may be affected in the average herd. It is estimated that the loss in yield in the subsequent lactation is about 14% and for those cows which have not died as a result of milk fever and a reduction in longevity. Very high levels of milk fever indicate that the management and feeding is wrong or there is a low magnesium intake or the animals have fatty liver. Most cases are seen between five and 10 years old and are at the time when the animals are producing their lifetime's peak lactations. More cases occur in the Channel Island breeds than most others. The condition does have an inherited component of about 6 to 12%. Milking out the cow in the first two days after calving will often precipitate the condition.

A few cases of milk fever are seen a day or two before calving, but most occur within 48 hours of the birth with a few up to 10 days afterwards. Very occasionally, the problem is seen at other times usually coinciding with bulling. High dietary concentrations of calcium at or around calving as the cause of milk fever has been questioned. In several studies in the USA, the overfeeding of calcium was only a problem when the levels of phosphorus were high and hypocalcaemia only occurred in a relatively narrow range of dietary concentrations of calcium (about 16 g Ca/kg DM) with either extreme concentrations of calcium being beneficial in the control of the disorder. The duration of feeding of extreme concentrations of calcium can, however, influence whether or not symptoms of hypocalcaemia develop.

6.4.1.1 Causal factors and signs

The problem of milk fever is one of mobilisation of calcium. If calcium levels are slightly low before calving than the system starts to prime itself to overcome this deficit. This means that vitamin D has to become activated (1,25 dihydroxyvitamin D) by undergoing changes in the liver and kidney. This more active form helps release parathyroid hormone from the parathyroid and this increases the absorption of calcium from the gut. Also, it causes resorption of calcium from the bones (osteoclastic remodelling) and reduces calcium loss in the urine. This mechanism is not fully understood but in practice diets containing less than 50g/Ca per day will lead to a negative balance of calcium whilst in use. The main reason for this is the demand of the cow and the developing calf exceeds the calcium supplied by the diet. Such diets are very difficult to achieve except with high cereals usage or one predominately of straw.

Magnesium is required to help in the activation of the vitamin D and also the parathyroid hormone and so when magnesium levels are low then the activation will not occur. Fatty liver is also associated with low magnesium levels and so again can result in milk fever problems. Diets with a high acidity can help to increase activation of the parathyroid hormone. This is the basis of DCAB - dietary cation-anion balance theory (see page 94).

The problem of milk fever is divided into three phases. In the first the cow becomes excitable with muscle tremors of the head and legs and teeth grinding. The temperature is normal and not raised as the name of the condition implies. The legs are stiff and the cow is not inclined to walk. She easily falls over with the legs stuck out stiffly. Often treatment at this stage is difficult and animals may not respond as well as expected.

The second phase is when the animal is resting on her brisket. She does not eat, drink, urinate or dung. The anus may be dilated and dung seen but not passed. She has a dry nose and mouth. The eyes are dilated, and the skin of the ears and legs feel cold. The temperature is low and the name milk fever is really a misnomer. The respirations increase in depth and there is usually a grunt or groan. The neck often develops a kink and in others the head is held into the side of the neck.

The third stage involves the cow going onto her side with the legs outstretched. If attempts are made to correct her position, the cow returns back onto her side. Often the animal will develop bloat. She is often very cold at this time and if untreated she will go into a coma and then die.

6.4.1.2 Treatment of the disorder

The standard treatment is calcium borogluconate and if this is to be given into the vein it must be done slowly. The standard bottle contains 400 or 500 ml of a 25% or 40% solution. Other calcium solutions can be used. These are usually more concentrated and so must be used with even greater care. The cow may also have the calcium given under the skin. This will usually not work on its own unless the cow is only showing a few signs and she is not down. It can however be used as an adjunct to intravenous treatment. The cow will initially have difficulty standing and will often lose her grip and damage herself. This can lead to a downer cow. Thus the animal should be kept at grass, or if indoors, the bedding should be allowed to build up so that the cow can gain some purchase for her feet. If the cow is down any length of time she will need to be turned. The cow should be allowed to rise in her own time and not be forced to try to rise. If she does try to stand then she should be supported so that she can be prevented from doing the splits. If the cow has hypomagnesaemia then this must also be treated.

6.4.1.3 Control and prevention of milk fever

Prevention is better than cure in the case of hypocalcaemia. It is essential to ensure that the cow is given a diet which will prime the absorption system. This involves the use of straw and some mineralised cereals or concentrates. At the end of pregnancy the diet can slowly be changed to the production ration. The level of concentrate feed offered should not be more than 3 or 4 kg DM. Some of the production roughage should also be offered. It is important to also maintain appetite and encourage eating. If problems have been bad the use of vitamin D or its analogues can be helpful. The use of oral dosing or intramuscular injections of vitamin D has been used successfully in the prevention and control of hypocalcaemia but the method requires an accurate prediction of date of calving. Repeated therapy using vitamin D can lead to toxicity. High doses of calcium chloride by mouth can also provide the right environment. The cow should not be milked out for the first few days after calving. The diet should be checked to make sure that it is not very alkaline as this can predispose to milk fever.

6.4.2 Hypomagnesaemia (Lactation Tetany)

The condition is complex but usually consists of a magnesium deficiency often with a concurrent mild calcium deficiency. Cattle require each day to receive the requirements of magnesium which are used in their maintenance and lactation. If this does not occur then blood magnesium levels rapidly fall (hypomagnesaemia) and signs of staggers may develop. Thus a short period of 24 to 48 hours starvation can precipitate the problem. Cattle are particularly susceptible in the month or so after calving although a more chronic form can often be seen in dry cows in the autumn.

In the early lactating cow the problem is usually seen in the spring when the cows are turned out onto lush rapidly growing pasture, particularly areas which have been fertilised with potash and, to a lesser extent, nitrogen. Often it follows a period of bad weather such as windy or rainy conditions which stress or chill the animals or frosts reducing feed intake and particularly where there is limited shelter for the animals. Many cows develop very loose faeces on spring pastures and this decreases transit time of feed through the gut and reduces absorption of magnesium and other nutrients. In the autumn problems arise where cows are at pasture with little or no supplementary feed and this leads to a slow and profound fall in the circulating magnesium levels and if the cow is then stressed, she will break down with the condition. Under such circumstances all animals in the same group will be hypomagnesaemic.

6.4.2.1 Signs

The signs of hypomagnesaemia are often very rapid in onset and an animal may graze normally, then stop and become intensely alert with muscle twitching. She may start to gallop around when slightly stimulated and also bellow. The gait becomes more and more staggery and the animal may fall over. She remains on her side and will have her head stretched over her back, she will often pass dung and urinate. The legs are held outstretched and she may be quiet. Then if she is stimulated at all she will stand working her legs as if she was running although on her side. This often digs up the earth under her legs, she will also be twitching and will froth at the mouth and again urinate and pass dung. The faeces are usually diarrhoeic. Often the heart can be heard beating away from the animal and the animal's temperature tends to be high. The cow can die in one of these periods of frenzied activity, and death is often within half to one hour of the animal going down.

A more chronic form can come on over a period of three or four days and the cow will be slightly off its feed and have a wild expression. In many instances when approached the cow weaves her neck about as if being hit. There are again muscle twitching and the animal may break down into the more severe form of the disease if she is stimulated. Sometimes, if the appetite returns the cow may get better. In the chronic winter form the animal has very vague signs with dullness, indifferent appetite, looses condition and may then develop the more usual form of the condition.

6.4.2.2 Treatment of the disorder

The treatment needs to be rapid and it must be remembered that even the stimulation of the cow by inserting a needle into her may lead to fatal convulsions. In some instances the veterinary surgeon will need to sedate the animal before trying any other form of therapy. The main form of therapy is to use magnesium which is given in the form of magnesium sulphate under the skin. This should provide relatively quick relief unless the animal has suffered brain darnage through its heightened activity and in such cases there may be a partial response but the animal remains excitable or very dull. The magnesium should not be injected into the vein as this can result in cardiac arrest and death. If it is thought necessary to give anything into the vein then calcium borogluconate should be administered slowly. This should be done by the veterinary surgeon.

6.4.2.3 Control and prevention

When problems of hypomagnesaemia are occurring it is necessary to increase the intake of feeds other than grass. Thus all cattle should receive and eat roughage after each milking and before being let out to pasture. Otherwise strip grazing to control intake can be helpful or the slow introduction to the pasture increasing the time allowed out each day. The use of permanent pasture will also produce less problems than new ones. Animals must have adequate shelter in case the weather is poor. If conditions become very cold or wet or windy the cattle should be rehoused until the weather improves. If problems occur every year and are associated with calving, then the calving season may need to be altered.

Feeding extra magnesium can be helpful. Most forms of magnesium are unpalatable and so need to be masked. Magnesium oxide is a cheap form of magnesium. This can be fed in silage or by supplying about 60 grams in a concentrate or mixed with molasses in a lick or block. Some forms of magnesium such as chloride or acetate can be added to the drinking water and can be successful, provided the cows do not reject the water or do not have access to other non treated sources. Magnesium can also be provided in the form of metal alloy bullets which provide a "top-up" over the first few weeks after their use.

The pastures can also be treated. Ideally the first pastures should not have had any potassium or nitrogen on them until after they have been grazed. Magnesium dusting of the pasture with fnely ground magnesium oxide or magnesium solution before turn out can work well. Otherwise the use of calcined magnesite or magnesium limestone as a fertiliser will help prevent the problem for a year or two.

6.5 Energy problems

All high yielding cows in early lactation will be unable to eat sufficient feed for the energy requirements of the milk which they will be producing. In early lactation the energy needs of a cow producing 30 litres a day are three times that required by the late pregnant animal. This energy gap is filled by mobilisation of fat and other body reserves of the cow resulting in a loss of weight and condition. The amount of this deficit will depend on the yield of the cow, the condition score of the cow at calving and how quickly the appetite improves so that the energy intake matches or exceeds the energy outputs. Usually the intake and loss balance out at about eight to 12 weeks after calving. The sooner this happens the better for the metabolism of the cow and the more likely she is not to suffer from other problems and diseases. The secret is thus to increase dry matter intake as quickly as possible after calving. The problems which can occur as a result of this energy lack can increase (Figure 6.1) from fatty liver syndrome (Section 6.5.1) to sub-clinical ketosis to ketosis (also called acetonaemia, Sections 6.5.2 and 6.5.3) to the very severe "fat cow" syndrome (Section 6.5.4).

Figure 6.1 Development of fat cow syndrome

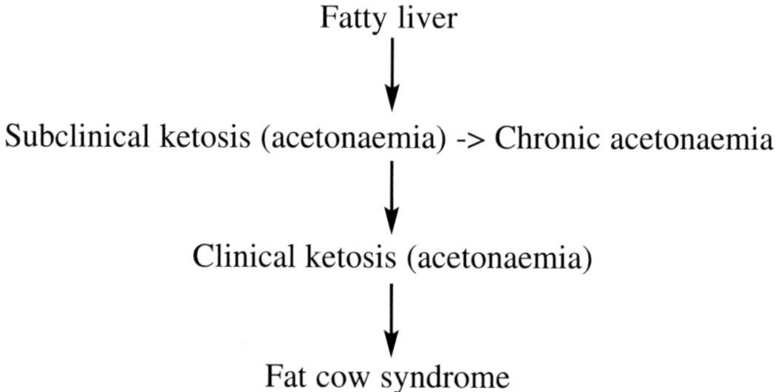

6.5.1 Fatty liver syndrome

As said above, inevitably cows will lose weight after calving to meet the energy deficit of their rations. This process is under the control of the endocrine system. This loss of condition will occur more in cows which do have a higher condition score at calving as their appetite will be slower to return to normal than thinner cows. The energy is provided by fat which is taken from its various stores such as under the skin, in the stomach cavity and around the kidney and heart and is transported to the liver in the blood plasma as free fatty acids (FFA).

Two fates of FFA could occur, the formation of so-called ketone bodies which are able to be used for energy production in the presence of some other energy substances produced from the diet or the synthesis of triglycerides (that is fat synthesised from the FFA). Fatty liver itself is thus not a disease but is a metabolic indicator of energy problems. The greater the energy deficiency, the more the fat is mobilised from its stores and in consequence the greater the building up of fat within the liver. This is the result of the liver having a lower capacity to secrete triglycerides than its ability to synthesis triglycerides.

During the first few days of lactation there is a marked increase in the level of fatty acids entering the liver. In a normal cow, these compounds are converted to cholesterol, other lipids and lipoproteins and used in the animal's energy metabolism. If however the liver contains large amounts of fat then it tends to become less efficient in its ability to deal with the fat accumulating within it as well as its other functions. This can then lead to acetonaemia which is a metabolic dysfunction but can relatively easily be treated.

Fat cow syndrome is uncommon but can often be fatal. Where any of these conditions are seen it is an indication that there is an energy deficiency problem in the herd and not just an individual animal. Thus the first one should be fully investigated as it is the early warning that there is something wrong in the dietary management of the herd.

6.5.1.1 Occurrence of fatty liver

The accumulation of fat in the liver affects the structure of the cells in the liver. A study which examined the ultrastructure of the liver showed that cows with livers containing less than 20% fat were normal, livers from cows with between 20 to 40% fat were classified at risk from metabolic problems and animals with over 40% of liver mass as fat were at significant risk from metabolic disorders.

Fatty liver is mainly seen in cows which are over-fat at calving, i.e. a condition score of over 3.0 or greater at calving. This occurs if the energy input in late lactation or the dry period has been too great and so has allowed accumulation of fat. This is an increased problem when cows are calving in the summer months and so are dry at grass in the spring or early summer when the grass is often lush and of high energy value. This increased fat is also within the body cavities, reducing space for the expansion of the stomachs and the intestines and thereby restricting appetite. The energy deficit is made up from the body reserves and this leads to excessive weight loss after calving. This in turn can lead to an increased incidence in metabolic, reproductive and infectious diseases.

6.5.1.2 The problem of fatty liver

Thus such animals have an increased risk of acetonaemia, as well as milk fever and hypomagnesaemia. The energy deficit at that time can also lead to poor nutritional supply to the eggs or ova which are developing within the ovaries and which will be the ones ovulated during the period when the cow is mated. This leads to an increase in the number of services to conception, an increased time before ovarian activity. There is also often an increase in the number of these animals which need to be culled as well as often they have a longer dry period. This latter problem is important in that a vicious circle can develop so that unless feeding is well controlled when dry the cow will once more be in too high a condition score and so develop fatty liver again. Fatty liver is usually a herd indication of high performance cows. The other problem can be an effect on the ability of the cow to deal with infectious disease. It appears that under the conditions of fatty liver the ability of the various cells in the blood and the body in general are less able to deal with infections and toxin production.

6.5.1.3 Control and prevention

The aim in controlling and preventing fatty liver is to ensure that cows are not in an excessive condition score before calving. The ideal is 2.5 to 3 and under these circumstances the appetite will increase relatively rapidly. It does mean that the condition of the cows must be watched in the second half of lactation so that the diet can be changed if the cow's condition starts to increase too much. In the dry period again it is essential not to feed more than for maintenance and pregnancy unless the animal is thin. It is very difficult to control feed intake while at grass and, if it is at a period of pasture growth, it is best to place them on a bare pasture or keep them inside. Very heavy stocking can also work.

The extent to which cows go off feed during the dry period is related to circulating non-esterified fatty acids and the accumulation of fats in the liver. Therefore if energy intake is maintained during the period immediately before calving, the reduction in fat accumulation in the liver in early lactation is minimised. Use of propylene glycol in the close up dry period may be one strategy to avoid fatty liver syndrome in dairy cows, however the benefits to milk production are not substantiated.

After calving the aim is to have high dry matter intakes in the first two weeks after calving. The milking diet should be fed in the last two weeks of the dry period but only at a level of about 3 to 4 kg DM so that the rumen organisms can become used to the new ration. While maintaining appetite the production ration should initially be mixed with more fibre and some less energy dense ration to try and not result in too large a change for the rumen. It is often best to keep the fresh calving cows separately so that they and their feed can be monitored better. Use of total mixed rations can be helpful to ensure good digestion as also can frequent small concentrate feeds or out of parlour feeders. Highly digestible forage should be available ad libitum. In addition there is a need to ensure that adequate supplies of protein are available including slowly degradable protein such as fishmeal or heated soyabean meal.

6.5.2 Acetonaemia

Acetonaemia, otherwise known as ketosis or slow fever, is the form of energy deficiency in which clinical signs develop. It can occur in any situation where there is a lack of energy. For practical purposes it is often divided into primary or secondary ketosis. The primary form is the result of the diet not providing sufficient energy. In the secondary form there is another problem which reduces the animal's appetite and so then causes the energy deficiency. Problems which can result in a secondary acetonaemia are legion, but some of the most common include mastitis, metritis, displacement of the abomasum, "wire" or traumatic reticulitis, peritonitis, and deficiencies such as phosphorus or cobalt.

The primary form can be subclinical and probably occurs to some extent in most high yielding cows, although the cow is able to compensate for this and thereby clinical signs do not develop. In the clinical form of the primary disease, the animal usually shows signs as her milk yield starts to rise. Thus most cases occur in the first month and especially in the 20 to 30 days after calving. It is less common in the south of England and particularly in the south west probably because these areas can produce more feed and the animals do not require so much energy to maintain warmth. Most problems arise in the winter period from October to April and especially following the start of the new year.

Various constituents of the diet are more likely to produce ketosis (ketogenic) than other parts. Thus the cereal part of the diet helps prevent the problem as does flaked maize. Hay is less ketogenic than grass silage. High protein diets produce more of the substances likely to cause acetonaemia.

6.5.2.1 Signs of acetonaemia

There are two main forms of the condition namely, the wasting and nervous forms. In the wasting form there is a gradual decrease in appetite and milk yield over a period of two to four days. There is an alteration in the choice of feed, with first concentrates being refused then grass silage and finally hay. Usually during and previous to this, the cow has been losing more weight than was to be expected. Often the dung is stiffer than its companions and the breath has a sweet pear drop, or acetone, smell to it, this can be smelled by some people but not others. The temperature, and breathing are normal and while the cow may appear otherwise normal, others are moderately depressed and some have a hang-dog expression and others appear blind and "star gaze".

The nervous form is usually observed by the onset suddenly of one or more nervous signs such as muscle twitching, over-excitable and often vigorous licking of the skin, walls and objects. Some appear blind or walk in circles or have a staggery gait or aimlessly wander. The nervous signs usually last for a period of a half to two hours and then return in another eight to 12 hours or so. However, usually the signs seen in the wasting form are also evident with alteration of appetite, loss of condition, hardened dung, normal temperature, and smell to the breath.

Neither of these forms of acetonaemia tend to be fatal but unless treated the yield is likely to be greatly decreased. The sooner the condition is diagnosed and treated the less damage is done to the lactation.

6.5.2.2 Treatment of acetonaemia

As the problem is one of energy deficiency, the aim of all therapy is to increase the amount of easily assimilated energy quickly. It is also essential to check that the problem is one of primary deficiency rather than secondary where some of the therapy would be inappropriate. Thus a veterinary surgeon diagnosis is essential and he will usually give the animal an injection of corticosteroids to increase and improve the efficiency of energy breakdown. This will often increase the milk yield depression for a few hours and also, in the nervous form, make the animal worse. Thus where there is the risk of complications or for a speedy relief some veterinary surgeons will give glucose intravenously with or without the corticosteroids. The use of drenches of energy producing substances may also be helpful and these include glycerol and propylene glycol. Sodium proprionate, sodium lactate and in the past chloral hydrate have all also been used. Flaked maize may also help tickle the palate.

6.5.2.3 Control and prevention

The key to the control of acetonaemia is feeding practice throughout the whole lactation and the dry period. Thus in the second half of lactation, provide a high proportion of fibre in the diet which can be of lower digestibility than peak yield and the feed should not be fed in excess of requirements. The animals should be condition scored so that at the start of the dry period they are at a condition score of 2.5 to 3. They must then be maintained at that condition score. In the last two weeks or so the same roughage should be given as will be fed in the early lactation. The animals should also in this period be given small quantities of the production ration. This can be slowly increased but this should not exceed more than 3 to 4 kg at calving. Overfeeding in this period can result in a reduced appetite initially after calving and increased condition loss.

After calving ideally the aim is to maintain appetite by providing good quality concentrates and slowly build up, equal to, or in advance of milk yield. All carbohydrates used should be easily digestible and have high quality protein in them including good levels of rumen undegradable protein plus adequate vitamins and minerals. Again the aim, often not achieved, is to have maximum dry matter intake at the same time as maximum yield. The concentrate should be fed a little and often, possibly using out of parlour feeders or as a total mixed ration. The roughage must remain good and the animals should receive enough exercise to allow good bodily function.

Ideally no changes in the ration should be made in the first three months of lactation. Where they must be made, all changes in constituents or batch of feed should be made gradually and ideally over 10 to 14 days. In the second three months the quantity of high quality concentrate should be reduced and more roughage introduced, but again all changes should be made gradually. Throughout lactation attention should be paid to the quality of the feeds and all feeds should be analysed for their nutritive value. It is always best to underestimate the nutritive value of the diet than overestimate it. Where there have been problems in silage quality e.g. butyric silage, moulding, or high free ammonia levels these must also be taken into account as they will radically reduce dry matter intake unless mixed with better quality materials.

6.5.3 Chronic acetonaemia

The majority of acetonaemia cases become better with treatment, however there are a small number which do not respond. In many instances this is because the treatment was too late or there was insufficient therapy or it was inappropriate. In some cases the animal is over-fat and so although it may temporarily respond, it will still not have sufficient appetite to meet its yield requirements. In other cases the therapy will work, but the animal will return to the diet which resulted in the problem in the first place and so the trouble will return.

Other reasons for a chronic problem are that the animal for whatever reason (a) has a reduced appetite, or (b) there is starvation, or (c) the animal is very high-producing.

6.5.3.1 Reduction in appetite

This can be just one animal which is usually too thin or too fat or a small cow. However the problem can be a herd one with the condition score in the herd being very variable with some cows too thin and some too fat at the same stage of lactation. In some herds it may be obvious that it is only the heifers which are affected. Usually the animals fail to reach their potential yield and there is a rapid decline in it. The cause of the reduced appetite and whether it is an individual or group problem needs to be determined. An increase in dietary fibre should be made and the cows encourage to eat more. Heifers should be kept separately to the cows.

6.5.3.2 Starvation

In this form of chronic ketosis, the animals are too thin. There is usually inadequate concentrate usage either in terms of its quality or quantity. In other cases the roughage, usually silage, is inadequate or of poor quality. Insufficient grass or again poor grass quality can be the cause. These cattle show a poor yield, with a low peak yield with a rapid fall-off and the milk protein percentage is low.

The control of the condition is to increase the quality and quantity of feed which is required. If grass is inadequate or of poor quality then buffer feeding should be introduced and the yield and condition score should be monitored.

6.5.3.3 High-yielding cows

In this form, there is a sharp fall in milk yield after calving. Usually the animals reach their peak yield at a very early stage after calving i.e. by two weeks. The peak yield is not maintained with again a rapid fall-off in yield and a sharp decrease in condition score after calving. The milk protein percentage is also lower. Often the animals will have had milk fever or swollen udders and, if a heifer, it is animals which are calving at about three years and probably in consequence have had too much feed at a time when they would have normally have been calved and milking. Often the feeding has included too high a concentrate usage in the dry period or heavy feeding early in lactation.

The aim is not to feed too much in the dry period and to encourage appetite to be maintained. After calving, the concentrate content of the ration should be slowly increased while encouraging the animal to eat.

6.5.4 Fat cow syndrome

There has been a lot of confusion about this problem as often it is called fatty liver syndrome. It is true that the condition does involve a fatty liver but unlike fatty liver syndrome, which is a normal physiological change in high yielding cows to the demands of milk production and produces no clinical signs, fat cow is an extreme condition which results in a high level of illness and often death. In addition while fatty liver syndrome is a common problem, fat cow syndrome is not. However it can become a herd problem if cattle are overfed in the last part of lactation and into the dry period. The condition is usually seen in cows rather than heifers and is more common when there is a long dry period. The condition became more common when increased milk prices encouraged summer calving. Thus cows became dry in the spring or early summer when grass was at its most plentiful and at its highest nutritional quality. If cattle were not severely restricted in their grazing or kept indoors then there was a tendency for them to receive too much energy for their requirements and so become fat. The signs of the condition occur soon after calving as a result of the sudden increase in energy demands in animals which cannot increase their appetites to meet them.

6.5.4.1 Signs of fat cow syndrome

The animals will calve in a condition score usually in excess of 4. Many of them will suffer milk fever. They will start to produce milk but will have a limited appetite and will rapidly lose weight. This results in a rapid loss of weight with severe acetonaemia which invariably does not or only partially responds to treatment. The animals are very prone to post calving infections such as mastitis or metritis and they tend not to respond to treatment or have a protracted response. The milk yield of the animals is poor and often they will only eat small quantities of feed or none at all. Many of the animals will become more and more ill until they become recumbent. Often they are constipated and pass only small quantities of hard dung, however as the condition progresses the dung may become diarrhoeic and very foul smelling. The coats are often dull with loss of hair and in some cases there is exudation onto the skin. Some animals will develop muscle twitching and other nervous signs. Those that survive will often not produce their anticipated milk yield and will also have fertility problems with a delay from calving to first service interval and more services before successful conception.

6.5.4.2 Treatment

This will first need a diagnosis by the veterinary surgeon and then the use of glucose producers in the form of intravenous glucose injections as well as probably corticosteroids. Often antibiotics will also be used to counteract any infections present or to prevent their occurrence. Treatment will need to be concentrated and often on a daily or alternate day basis. The animals must be encouraged to eat and this will often involve tempting them with different types of feed. The use of flaked maize can also be useful.

6.5.4.3 Prevention

The problem can arise one year and then if the animal takes longer to become pregnant, their dry periods increase and so more cases occur unless remedial measures are taken. The control measures for acetonaemia also control fat cow syndrome. The most important procedures are to control the diet in the second half of lactation so that the cows are dried off at a condition score of 2.5 to 3.

However the problem is often on a herd basis and by the time it is diagnosed other cattle are already dry and in a too fat state. If the cattle with the condition are becoming very ill and some are dying or requiring casualty slaughter, then it might be necessary to undertake some drastic measures. These are not without some risk and will need to be carefully monitored as well as involving your veterinary surgeon and nutrition adviser.

The aim is to place the cattle on a slimming diet. This should only be done where the condition of each animal is monitored and recorded to determine the weight loss. The aim is to provide as low energy diet as possible and to allow the cow to lose weight and break down her body reserves in an efficient way. The diet is based on straw plus a source of undegradable protein, usually fish meal which is fed at a level of 0.25 to 0.5 kg per day. The high calcium of this diet is counteracted by a low calcium high phosphorus mineral/ vitamin mix.

The animals should be given exercise so that they can utilise their diets more effectively. Usually cattle start to lose weight after two or three weeks on the diet, but this rate of loss is very variable and hence the need to condition score the individual animals at least once a fortnight and, when weight loss is occurring, every week. Some animals will not lose weight for a considerable time but then will rapidly lose it and these need to be monitored every few days.

The diet can continue unless there is very rapid weight loss until two weeks before calving when it must be replaced by one similar to that for acetonaemia prevention with the use of three to four kg dry matter of the production ration including the usual vitamin and mineral supplements, the introduction of some of the production forage and probably still some straw. The animals must still receive adequate exercise. After calving the production ration should be slowly increased so that the animals maintain their appetite.

6.6 Left displaced abomasum

Left displaced abomasum is becoming seen increasingly in high-yielding cows. Most cases are detected within six weeks of calving although they may not always be that easily diagnosed. The condition is usually seen in cattle on diets with a high cereal content and limited fibre intake particularly of long length. More cases are seen in the autumn and winter, but this may be due to a concentration of calvings at that time. Other factors which may be involved include a change in the acid-base balance at calving. Thus in the spring at grass the balance becomes more acidic but this alters to a more alkaline direction from late summer into the winter period. Other forms of organ swelling or twisting can be seen, but they are less common. Most result from the presence of highly fermentable feeds, such as cereals, not being digested in the rumen and so entering parts of the gut where they would not normally occur. This allows them to undergo an abnormal digestive process where gas is formed and can distend or misplace parts of the gut.

6.6.1 Causes

The problem is thought to be due to an excess of the volatile fatty acids which are produced by the digestion of grain entering the abomasum rather than being absorbed through the rumen wall. This leads to the abomasum losing its muscle tone and becoming enlarged and flabby. The organ can then move about more freely within the abdomen (stomach cavity). The recent calving will mean that there is relatively more space in the abdomen following the loss of the calf, the foetal fluids and the placenta. Thus the now more mobile abomasum can become trapped under the rumen. As the blood supply is not affected the signs are those of a digestive type. In long standing cases, complications can occur such as abomasal ulceration and localised peritonitis.

6.6.2 Signs

The signs are usually within a few days or a week of calving, the cow has a reduced appetite with milk yield not being as expected and a variable degree of acetonaemia. Often the animal will eat one day and on the next she will only pick at her feed. The left side of the animal when viewed from the back may appear to go straight down rather than be more rounded. The temperature and breathing rate normal. The dung is usually softer than the other cows or at times diarrhoeic. Gas is usually entrapped in the abomasum and can be heard as characteristic sounds on the left side of the abdomen by your veterinary surgeon.

6.6.3 Treatment

Very occasionally there is spontaneous recovery, but most animals will require treatment. This can be in the form of casting and rolling the cow. This can be successful in some cases and the animal must then be placed on a hay or straw diet without concentrates for several days before concentrates are re-introduced. However rolling is often unsuccessful or the abomasum may retum to its correct position only to again become displaced. In consequence cattle with the condition are often operated upon. There are many different approaches to the surgery, but once the abomasum is repositioned, the abomasum is usually anchored to the muscles forming the wall of the abdomen. Following surgery, the cow must again be kept on a high roughage diet for several days before the slow introduction of concentrates.

6.6.4 Prevention

It is important to try and keep the gut working properly during the calving period and the cow should be offered and must eat some long fibre roughage. Concentrate introduction in the dry period should be limited and then after calving they should only be slowly increased. Practices such as steaming up cows should be avoided.

Further recommended reading

Andrews, A.H., Blowey, R.W., Boyd, H. and Eddy, R.G. (1992) *Bovine Medicine*. Blackwell Sciences Ltd. Oxford, UK.

Andrews, A.H. (2000) *The Health of Dairy Cattle*. Blackwell Sciences Ltd. Oxford, UK.

McClure, T.J. (1994) *Nutritional and Metabolic Infertility in Cattle.* CAB International, Wallingford, UK.

Chapter 7
FUTURE PROSPECTS

The management of the expectant dairy cow, particularly during the six to eight weeks of the dry period has to be precise in order to ensure the animal is fit for the onset of lactation. The management regime applied to the cow has to encompass issues of behaviour, nutrition, health and welfare. If progress is to be made in the development of a blue-print for the dry period several key questions have to be addressed and answered. If these questions are not investigated the management of the dry cow may not ensure optimal economic output from the dairy system.

7.1 Welfare, health and issues concerned with social behaviour

The complex issues concerning social behaviour of cows during late lactation, the early dry period and the close-up dry period has to be investigated further. If a stable social hierarchy is produced amongst mature cattle, the status of the pregnant heifer or first lactation cow has to be examined. The pregnant heifer or first lactation cow, if housed with mature cows, may not be able to compete for feed and therefore concern over poor nutrition could be raised as an issue. The principles of good welfare (freedom from hunger, thirst, pain, heat, cold and sickness) must be applied to the housing, feed trough allocation and grouping of animals. It is important to recognise that a cow in late pregnancy may suffer from malnutrition as a result of poor development of social hierarchy or the inability of the cow to acquire adequate levels of nutrient to sustain foetal growth and development while not compromising the storage of nutrients as body reserves. Until relatively recently, the dry cow has been "neglected" as she requires a low level of nutrients and has been viewed as an animal who can sustain herself on minimal inputs of direct labour. However the development of "elite" herds and an increased perception of the general public towards the management of animals in agricultural systems as lead to a re-appraisal of the situation.

The rapid increase in the rate of genetic progress in recent times has lead to a serious challenge to farmers and producers of milk. In the situation where "elite" cows are managed with "average" cows, a certain degree of neglect or poor management practice may occur. This is not to say that the herdsman is not being precise about the management of the herd, but the obvious fact that these cows may need different nutritional management programmes during late lactation and pregnancy leads to the inevitable conclusion of neglect in certain circumstances. Ways and means to overcome these problems using simple systems must be applied. Complex answers of grouping or sub-grouping of animals for certain periods of the production cycle are not likely to work in practice or use substantially higher levels of labour that can be supported by the output of the herd. Optimisation of the chosen system should be based on benefit:cost relationships for animal welfare as well as economic benefit.

Genetic progress can be further accelerated by the use of biotechnology. The application of new technologies may lead to several problems during the dry period and potentially during the period immediately after parturition. Welfare implications of any process of unconventional breeding must be examined closely, for instance the development of systems that lead to oversize foetus, the impact of twinning on the requirement for extra nutrients during the dry period and any potential health problems that may be associated with the production of the calf. It could be suggested that better management of "traditional" methods of breeding and animal improvement (for example artificial insemination) should be examined in relation to our current knowledge of the dry period.

7.2 Nutrition

Our understanding of the detailed requirements of the cow during the dry period is still relatively poor. The old adage that a good start to a lactation is the result of precise management of the cow during the later stages of the previous lactation and the dry period is important, especially in the case of cows yielding more than 10000 litres.

Nutrition of the cow is not just concerned with the supply of nutrients to ensure her requirements for energy, protein and minerals are met, but it is also associated with the development of feed characterisation systems. Any application of a nutritional blue-print has to be developed on the basis of accurate methods to predict the actual nutrient values of feeds offered.

The system used in the United Kingdom to predict the energy requirement of dry cows is based on a series of factorial experiments and therefore the match of dietary input of energy to the dietary requirements is estimated, without consideration of social behaviour or modifications of ingestive behaviour. The major weaknesses in the current system are its inability to respond to abrupt changes in requirement and to adequately quantify the contribution made from the mobilisation of body reserves. The problem in the quantification of energy derived from tissue mobilisation is especially important in the management of cows that are too fat in the late dry period and the management of the cow given diets that contain high levels of DUP to manipulate the maternal protein store. What are the costs associated with the development of maternal protein stores and the cost of maintaining those stores during periods of rapid foetal growth? Furthermore little is know about the true costs (in energy terms) of repair and development of new secretory tissue in the quiescent mammary gland.

It must also be noted that the methods of characterisation of substrates which make up the metabolisable energy are relatively unsophisicated. Clearly it is inadequate to continue to develop systems of evaluation which are detached from studies made with the cow herself. At present there is a potential risk of over-estimating the nutrient values of feeds offered to the dry cow and little or no quantification of the energy yield from for instance amino acids available for foetal utilsation.

The method of scoring the condition of cows during the dry period is a practical approach to ensure the nutrition of the cow is adequate. This method is relatively sensitive to changes in fat (energy) stores, but not adequate to assess the maternal protein store. A further refinement of the method must be made. For instance can an assessment of maternal protein store be made by examination of the biceps femoris (hock to pin) ?

The link between the energy and protein systems used in practical rationing of the dairy cow in all stages of production is the concept of fermentable metabolisable energy or the energy available from feeds to optimise the synthesis of microbial protein. There are to date no accurate measures of fermentable metabolisable energy. The concept also is flawed as it does not consider the yield of energy from the fermentation of amino acids. Therefore the estimation of metabolisable protein for cows during the dry period may be inadequate and lead to a restriction in supply of amino acids to the developing foetus. The main effect of this situation would be a reduction in birth weight and potentially a reduced likelihood of survival of the calf during the early neonate stage.

No consideration in diet formulation has been made of the impact of the cows labile protein reserves. The existence of these reserves actually reduces the effects of inadequate formulation. Foetal metabolism, especially during the late stages of pregnancy relies increasingly on the supply of amino acids as an energy source. Mobilisation or modification of the maternal protein stores may well prevent malnutrition of the foetus, but the long-term effect of poor management may be a reduction in the potential production of milk and reproductive performance of the cow during the early phases of the subsequent lactation. Further information is necessary to ensure the requirements for protein during the close-up dry period are fulfilled.